Principles of
Acute
Coronary
Care

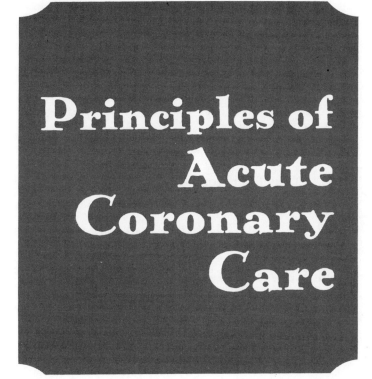

Principles of Acute Coronary Care

William T. Foster, M.D.

Director, Coronary Care Unit
Howard Memorial Hospital
Willits, California

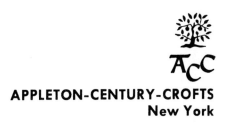

APPLETON-CENTURY-CROFTS
New York

FOREWORD

This book has been written out of pure necessity. A number of years ago, when I began giving lectures in acute coronary care, there were no textbooks available on the subject. Consequently, I relied on handouts made on the office copying machine, material from drug companies, and pamphlets from the American Heart Association. None of these publications gave a complete resume of the information needed by the acute coronary care nurse or physician.

I rationalized that if I waited a few years, someone would come out with a good text on the subject of Acute Coronary Care. None has. So now, even though I am not a cardiologist, I have found it necessary to put into a concise form, the basic material needed by both physicians and nurses who assume coronary care. By so doing, I trust that I will not affront my cardiologist friends who have contributed immeasurably to this publication.

The information contained herein is not meant to provide all the current knowledge or concepts involved with acute coronary care. One must go to the journals, as I have done, to appreciate the constant flux of opinion and ideas which currently make up "acute coronary care". The coronary care unit is barely ten years old, and during this time we have learned more about the acute coronary patient than in all the previous history of medicine. We have attempted to put this knowledge into an easily readable form and offer it as a handy reference manual for the standard and accepted concepts of acute coronary care.

It is hoped that this publication will be revised at regular intervals to keep up with new developments and procedures.

I sincerely hope that the reader of this book gets as much from it as has the author.

W. T. Foster, M. D.

DEDICATION

This book is respectfully dedicated to those poor lonely souls on the 11 to 7 shift who sit for hours with one eye on the monitor and the other eye on their arrhythmia manual.

CONTENTS

CHAPTER 1

ANATOMY OF THE HEART

A.   EXTERNAL ANATOMY

The heart sets in the anterior inferior mediastinum, weighs approximately 600 grams in the normal adult, and is roughly the size and configuration of the right hand made into a fist. It consists of four chambers (the right atrium and ventricle and the left atrium and ventricle) and is divisible into three layers. The inner layer, or endocardium, lines the chambers and is very thin. The middle layer, the myocardium, is the cardiac muscle and accounts for most of the mass of the heart. The outer layer is the epicardium and is also quite thin. A thick fibrous sheath, called the pericardium, covers about two-thirds of the heart surface.

The anterior aspect of the heart, that is, the surface of the heart viewed as if the anterior, or front, chest wall was completely transparent is seen in Figure 1.1. Structures to note are the superior vena cava (SVC), inferior vena cava (IVC), right atrium (RA), right ventricle (RV), pulmonary arteries (PA), pulmonary veins (PV), left ventricle (LV), and the aorta (AO).

The posterior aspect of the heart (the back surface) consists primarily of the left atrium (LA) and left ventricle (LV) as seen in Figure 1.2. Other structures to note are the inferior vena cava, superior vena cava, right atrium, pulmonary artery, pulmonary veins and the aorta.

1

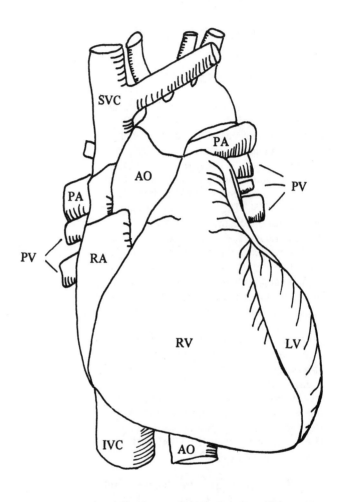

Figure 1.1   The anterior aspect of the heart.

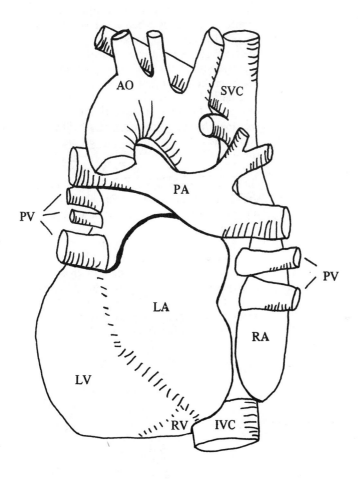

Figure 1.2   The posterior aspect of the heart.

3

The majority of the anterior surface of the heart and approximately one-half of the posterior surface is covered by the pericardium.

The external anatomy of the heart is of interest clinically when we view the chest X-ray. The routine PA (posterior-anterior; the front surface of the chest flush against the X-ray film with the X-ray machine shooting from the back) view of the chest is shown diagrammatically in Figure 1.3 with the parts of the heart outline. Of significance is the fact that the right side of the heart silhouette is the right atrium and the left sided silhouette is the left ventricle. No other chambers are seen on the PA X-ray of the chest. The pulmonary artery and aorta can usually be distinguished and any enlargement of either structure detected on the PA film.

Two other X-ray views which are useful in determining enlargement of chambers or structures are the right anterior oblique and the left anterior oblique. Figures 1.4 and 1.5 are diagrams of these two views and show the structures to be noted.

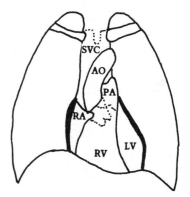

Figure 1.3   Posterior-Anterior (PA) view of the heart.

4

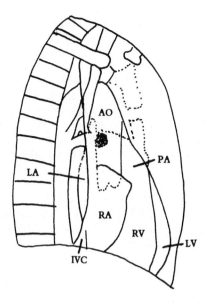

Figure 1.4   Right anterior oblique view of
the heart.

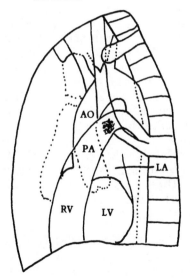

Figure 1.5   Left anterior oblique view of
the heart.

5

B.   INTERNAL ANATOMY

As a summary of the internal anatomy of the heart, one can readily trace the flow of blood through the various chambers and valves. Refer to Figure 1.6. The blood from the upper extremities, head and neck comes back to the heart by way of the superior vena cava entering the right atrium. Blood from the lower extremities and abdomen feed into the right atrium from the inferior vena cava. The chemical content of the blood from the inferior vena cava is frequently different from that in the superior vena cava. In the right atrium, the two are mixed and can be referred to as mixed venous blood.

From the right atrium, the blood passes through the tricuspid valve into the right ventricle. The next contraction of the ventricle forces the blood through the pulmonic valve into the pulmonary artery. The venous blood may then go either into the right or left pulmonary artery. After traversing the pulmonary capillary bed, where gaseous exchange takes place, the blood then passes back to the heart through the pulmonary veins into the left atrium. The schematic drawing on Figure 1.6 shows one pulmonary vein from each lung. Actually the left lung generally has three pulmonary veins and the right lung two.

From the left atrium, the blood passes through the mitral valve into the left ventricle. The next contraction forces the blood through the aortic valve into the aorta and the general circulation.

The atria are separated by the interatrial septum and the ventricles by the interventricular septum. Note that the wall of the left ventricle is thicker than the right. This has to do with the fact that the left

6

ventricle must sustain a much higher blood
pressure than the right.

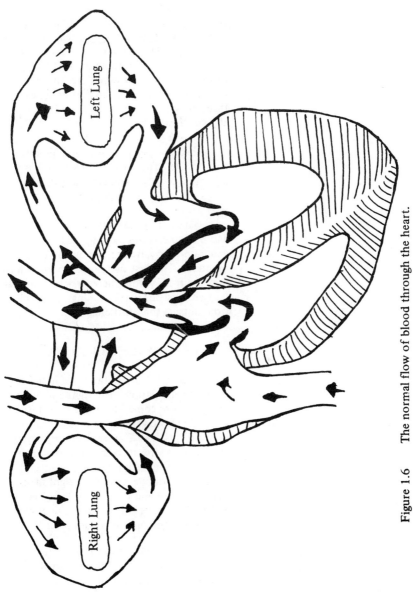

Figure 1.6   The normal flow of blood through the heart.

Figure 1.7 is a diagrammatic representation of the mitral or tricuspid valves. Each valve cusp is attached to a papillary muscle by cord-like fibrous structures called chordae tendineae and each of the chordae tendineae from a single papillary muscle extends to two valve cusps. There are usually three valve cusps per valve with three papillary muscles (sometimes two and sometimes more than three). Note that the papillary muscles arise from the wall of the ventricle and are actually contiguous with that wall.

Figure 1.8 represents the pulmonic or aortic valve. These two valves are referred to as semilunar valves and are made up of three cusps but without any attachments.

The difference in structure of the mitral and tricuspid valves as compared to the aortic and pulmonic valves can be explained by their function. The first two must support a high pressure from within the ventricle. The latter two must support a less high pressure from outside the ventricle.

C.   CORONARY CIRCULATION

Figure 1.9 shows the usual mode of the coronary circulation. The right and left coronary arteries come off of the aorta just beyond the aortic valve in an area called the sinus of Valsalva. The left coronary artery divides soon after its origin into two main branches; the anterior descending artery which sends out vessels to the right main bundle branch and the circumflex artery which goes posteriorly to anastamose with branches of the right coronary artery.

The right coronary artery sends a small branch anteriorly called the marginal artery. Its major branches extend posteriorly around the heart and by the posterior descending

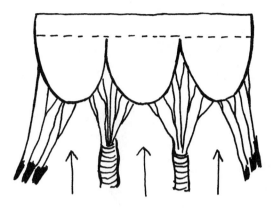

Figure 1.7   Tricuspid or mitral valve dissected and spread longitudinally.

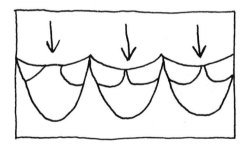

Figure 1.8   Pulmonic or aortic valve dissected and spread longitudinally.

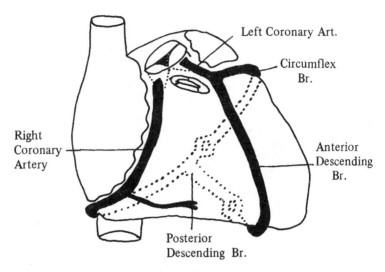

Figure 1.9   The Coronary Circulation

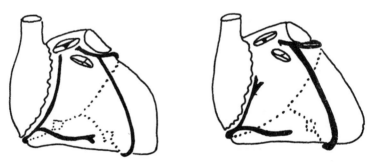

Figure 1.10   Figure 1.11

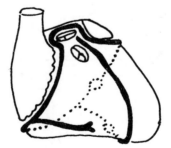

Figure 1.12

branch supplies the AV node, Bundle of His, and the left main bundle branch.

The vascular supply to the SA node comes off the proximal right coronary artery in about 55% of hearts and from the proximal left circumflex in about 45%.

There are three major deviations in the anatomy of the coronary circulation. Figure 1.10 shows the posterior descending branch of the coronary circulation coming off the circumflex branch of the left coronary artery. In Figure 1.11 there is but one coronary artery supplying the entire epicardial surface. Figure 1.12 shows the circumflex branch being off the right coronary artery rather than the left.

It is important to realize that the coronary vessels are perfused (the blood flows through them) only during diastole (the resting phase of the cardiac cycle).

D.   MYOCARDIUM

The myocardium is the cardiac muscle and is responsible for all the work of the heart. The muscle bundles of the myocardium are distributed in a circular fashion around the heart. See Figure 1.13.

E.   CONDUCTION SYSTEM OF THE HEART

This subject will be dealt with in a later chapter.

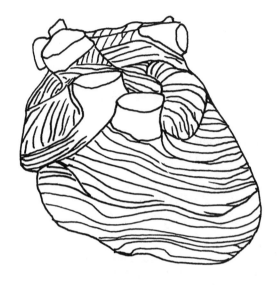

Figure 1.13   Myocardial bundles.

CHAPTER 2

PHYSIOLOGY OF THE HEART

A. PRIMARY PHYSIOLOGIC PROP-
    ERTIES

   There are three physiologic properties
of cardiac tissue:
      1.   Automaticity (rhythmicity)
      2.   Conductivity
      3.   Contractility
We will consider the first two (automaticity
and conductivity) in a later chapter dealing
with arrhythmias.

   The contractility of the heart is by virtue of the myocardium being a true muscle.
The myocardial muscle fibers however, un-
like other muscle fibers in the body, exhibit
an "all or none" response to stimulation.
For example, the biceps in the arm may be
contracted to 50% of its ability, held for an
indefinite period of time, then relaxed, or
contracted even more fully. Cardiac muscle
is unable to perform in such a manner. When
cardiac muscle fibers contract they do so immediately to their fullest extent. A cardiac
contraction can be sustained for only a fraction of a second and the myocardium then
relaxes automatically.

B.   PRIMARY PHYSIOLOGIC FUNCTIONS

   The primary functions of the heart are
actually two in number. It is a pump to
maintain:
      1.   Blood pressure and peripheral
           blood flow.
      2.   Perfusion of the lungs.

13

We may sum up all the functions of the heart by simply referring to cardiac output.

Let us consider what happens during the normal cardiac cycle. Referring to Figure 1.6 again trace the course of blood through the heart. Blood enters the right atrium from the superior and inferior vena cava, goes through the tricuspid valve into the right ventricle. It then goes past the pulmonic valve into the main pulmonary artery, and then either to the right or left pulmonary artery into the right or left lung. It returns to the heart through the pulmonary veins into the left atrium, through the mitral valve to the left ventricle, and finally out through the aortic valve into the aorta.

C.   INTRACARDIAC PRESSURES

Pressures within the heart chambers and great vessels during the normal cardiac cycle are of some significance. In the superior vena cava (which is synonymous with the central venous pool) the normal pressure is greater than 5 and less than 15cm of water, with a mean pressure of 7cm H_2O, or 5mm of mercury. Note that there are two ways to measure these pressures — cm of water or mm of mercury (Hg). All pressures within the heart are expressed in mm Hg. As would be expected, the pressure in the right atrium is essentially the same as the central venous pressure (5mm Hg). After the blood passes through a valve (in this case, the tricuspid valve), the pressure gradient normally rises and we can begin measuring both the systolic and diastolic pressures. In the right ventricle the normal systolic pressure is 30 mm Hg and the diastolic pressure 5mm Hg. As the blood passes through another valve, the pulmonic, the systolic pressure must remain the same, and indeed is found to be 30mm Hg. Because the pulmonic valve prevents full emptying of the pulmonary artery, the diastolic pressure drops to only 12 mm Hg.

14

When we measure the central venous 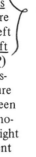 pressure or right atrial pressure what we are really interested in knowing is the mean left atrial pressure, which is the same as the left ventricular end-diastolic pressure (LVEDP) (the filling pressure), and we attempt to estimate this from the central venous pressure or right atrial pressure. However, it has been found that in several disease states, most notably early left heart failure, the CVP or right atrial pressure does not accurately represent the LVEDP. The mean left atrial pressure and LVEDP can be more accurately measured by means of the Swan-Ganz catheter. This is also called a PA (Pulmonary artery) line. It is a small calibre polyethylene tube with a double lumen. It is passed, just like the central venous catheter, into the superior vena cava, and right atrium. A small rubber bulb at the tip of the catheter is then inflated with air and the tip allowed to float through the left ventricle and into the pulmonary artery. The tip is then advanced into a small branch of the pulmonary artery until it is wedged. This is called the wedge pressure and is a true measurement of the mean left atrial pressure and LVEDP, and is the most sensitive indicator at the present time of incipient heart failure.

Whether one uses the CVP or the wedge pressure, it is important to understand that the initial reading is not the significant figure – unless, of course, it is exceedingly high or low – but rather, the changes in the pressure. This pressure should be monitored closely during volume load, during fluid therapy or during the acute phase of the patient's illness. Refer to Table 1 for a summary of the above-mentioned pressures.

Mention should also be made of the fact that with chronic pulmonary vascular

15

disease (as in pulmonary hypertension) even the wedge pressure is unreliable.

	Upper Normal Limits				During Fluid Therapy Do Not Exceed			
	cm H_2O		mm Hg		cm H_2O		mm Hg	
	S/D	Mean	S/D	Mean	S/D	Mean	S/D	Mean
CVP*		7		5		20		15
Right Atrium*		7		5		20		15
Right Ventricle			30/5					
Pulmonary Artery			30/12	25				
Wedge*		16		12		27		20
Left Atrium		16		12		27		20
LVED	16		12					

*Commonly measured

Table 1.   Intracardiac Pressures

The equipment necessary to determine the CVP includes a central venous catheter and a simple water manometer. Minimal skill is needed by the physician for the insertion of the catheter. To determine the wedge pressure, one needs a Swan-Ganz catheter, pressure transducer, and a monitor channel. Some additional skill is required to insert the Swan-Ganz.

D. THE CARDIAC CYCLE

If pressure sensitive instruments are placed in the left atrium, left ventricle, and aorta and the pressures recorded through a cardiac cycle the result is the graph seen in Figure 2.1. A simultaneous recording of the electrocardiogram and phonocardiogram is included in the graph. The pressure graph is calibrated from zero to 120mm Hg.

Note that prior to systole (the contraction phase of the cardiac cycle) the pressure in the left atrium is greater than that in the left ventricle. With the onset of systole there is closure of the mitral valve, which is represented by the intersection of lines LA and LV, and the left ventricular pressure rises. The period of rise from closure of the mitral valve to the point where the LV pressure line intersects with the aortic line is called the period of isometric contraction.

In diastole (the resting phase of the cardiac cycle) (Figure 2.2) the blood flows directly from the pulmonary veins into the left atrium and through the mitral valve into the left ventricle. Systole is divided into the isometric phase, noted above, (Figure 2.3) and the expulsion phase (Figure 2.4). During the isometric contraction phase the ventricle has contracted forcefully enough to close the mitral valve but not forcefully enough to

17

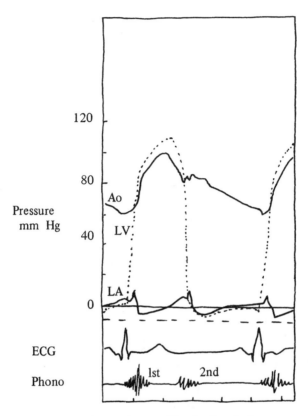

Pressure
mm Hg

120

80

40

0

Ao

LV

LA

ECG

Phono

1st   2nd

Figure 2.1   The Cardiac Cycle

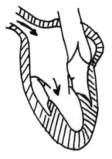

Fig. 2.2
Diastole

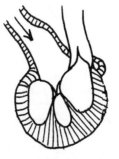

Fig. 2.3
Systole
Isometric
Contraction

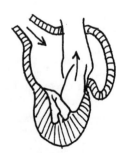

Fig. 2.4
Systole
Expulsion
Phase

expel blood through the aortic valve.

Referring back to Figure 2.1, at the intersection of the aortic and LV pressure lines the aortic valve opens and blood is then forced through the valve into the aorta by the contracting ventricle. Note the similarity in the pressure measurements of the LV and aorta. As the ventricle relaxes and the pressure drops the pressure lines intersect again and this represents closure of the aortic valve. During the expulsion phase (Figure 2.4) note that the aortic valve is wide open. Also note that during this phase of systole the atrium is already in full diastole and being filled by blood.

The pressures in both the atrium and ventricle go below the zero line into an area of negative pressure which enhances diastolic filling. In the graph, the aortic pressure never goes below 60mm Hg and represents a normal peripheral blood pressure.

Corresponding changes on the electrocardiogram are noted. The phonocardiogram shows the placement of the heart sounds in the cardiac cycle. The first heart sound is caused by closure of the AV valves (mitral & tricuspid), vibration of blood through the aortic valve, and vibration of blood through the chordae tendineae and fibers on the wall of the ventricle. The first sound usually occurs just after the end of the R wave on the ECG.

The second heart sound is caused by closure of the aortic and pulmonic valves and occurs just after the T wave. There is an often described but seldom heard third heart sound which is due to rapid filling of blood from the atrium into the ventricle.

Important points to remember are that the heart fills during diastole and that the

19

coronary vessels are perfused during diastole. The cardiac cycle is observed clinically by the electrocardiogram.

A pressure recording of the right side of the heart during the cardiac cycle could be obtained in a similar fashion. The results would be very similar to those obtained above. The only difference would be in the magnitude of the pressure gradients — which are obviously lower in the right side of the heart. The ECG and phonocardiogram recordings would be exactly the same.

E.   CARDIAC RESERVES

When the heart is fulfilling its functions, even in the face of increased demands, we say that it is in compensation or compensated. When it is not fulfilling these functions in the face of increased demands, we say that it is decompensated. Factors which allow the heart to compensate when faced with increased demands are called cardiac reserves. The cardiac reserves are essentially three in number.

1.   INOTROPHIC RESERVE
The first reserve of cardiac function lies in the increased strength of the cardiac contractions. This is called positive inotropism, and is under direct control of sympathetic nervous system stimulation. Adrenergic drugs can likewise produce this kind of response. The net effect of this kind of stimulation is an increase in stroke volume and thus in cardiac output. This happens by the working of three different mechanisms. Referring again to Figure 2.1 it is noted that if the time of systole is shortened and the heart rate remains the same then the diastolic filling time will increase. Of course, the amount of diastolic filling will likewise increase, and this is exactly what happens.

20

More complete emptying is also achieved by more forceful contractions, and this allows for quicker filling by increasing the negative pressure and resultant suction effect. Thirdly, sympathetic stimulation causes an augmented atrial contraction which produces an increased fiber length at the end of diastole in the ventricles. The importance of this will be considered later.

The natural long term effect of the increased strength of cardiac contractions, as seen for instance in hypertension, is cardiac hypertrophy. In this condition the heart enlarges mainly by increasing the amount of myocardium. Just as when an individual exercises muscles by weight lifting, these muscles get larger. In a similar way the cardiac muscle gets larger. There is a limit to which this process can go, however. The nutritional needs of any cell increase by the cubic volume of the cell, whereas the ability to supply nutrients to the cell increases only as the surface area. Therefore, hypertrophy of the heart is a self-limited process and may eventually lead to another condition called dilatation, which is a form of decompensation. All that has been mentioned concerning hypertrophy of the heart is assuming that the venous pressure remains normal. Should it increase, other processes become involved.

2.   INCREASED VENOUS PRESSURE

The second reserve of cardiac function has to do with the fact that increased venous filling pressure in the atrium will increase cardiac output. This is also under sympathetic nervous system control. In order to understand this phenomenon we must look to Starling's Law of the Heart. This is one of the most significant natural laws having to do with cardiac function. Refer to Figure 2.5. Starling's original hypothesis was that the stroke volume depends on the end diastolic stretch. The stroke volume can be equated roughly to cardiac output (in liters

21

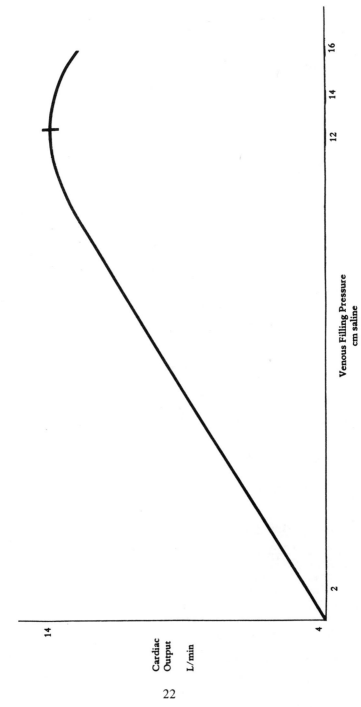

Figure 2.5   Starling's Law of the Heart

22

per minute) and the end diastolic stretch can
be equated to venous filling pressure. Looking at Figure 2.5 one can see that as the venous
filling pressure increases from zero to 12-13cm
of water (or saline) that the cardiac output increases to a maximum of about 14 liters per
minute. However, as the venous pressure continues to rise (that is, above 13cm of water)
an area of decompensation is reached and the
cardiac output drops.

This process of increased venous pressure leading to increased cardiac output can
be secondary to sympathetic stimulation
through venoconstriction, which, in turn, leads
to increased venous pressure. This is a natural
form of cardiac reserve. Increased venous pressure can also be achieved by increasing the
blood volume by infusion of intravenous
fluids.

3.   CHRONOTROPIC RESERVE
The third and final method by which
the heart may compensate by increased cardiac
output from sympathetic stimulation is simply
by an increased heart rate. This is true however, only if the filling pressure remains constant. Increased heart rate will raise the cardiac output only to a limit of about 180 beats
per minute. It must be recognized that increased heart rate also means increased oxygen consumption by the myocardium, and at
about 180 beats per minute the myocardium
has reached the point of diminishing returns
as far as oxygen consumption is concerned.

F.   CARDIAC OUTPUT

Natural changes in the cardiac output
are seen in a number of situations. The CO
will decrease with prolonged immobile standing, and can do so to the point of syncope.
This is why soldiers faint after standing at
attention for a long time. There is a decrease

in cardiac output with any damage to the heart. This means that with any degree of myocardial infarction, no matter how small, there will be a definite decrease in the cardiac output. At one time this was felt not to be true, but is now well established. The cardiac output will increase with the ingestion of food or even water. Naturally, it will increase with exercise. It will also increase with hypoxia (decreased oxygen in the blood) and in weather cold enough to cause shivering.

Originally, cardiac output was measured according to the Fick Method. This method simply states that the CO can be determined by the measurement of the volume of gas in venous as compared to arterial blood, and can be expressed by the following formula:

$$CO = \frac{O_2 \text{ Used}}{\text{A-V } O_2} \text{ or } \frac{CO_2 \text{ Produced}}{\text{A-V } CO_2}$$

This appears to be a simple method (that is, measuring the oxygen or carbon dioxide content of arterial and venous blood). In fact this is a difficult measurement to perform without rather sophisticated instruments to do so. In some of the larger medical centers, another method called the Dye Dilution Technique is used. By this method, a dye is injected into the venous circulation and is then measured in the arterial circulation. Again, this sounds like a simple technique but requires the use of a computer programmed to extrapolate the results of the blood measurements.

In everyday clinical practice several methods are used to estimate cardiac output. One of these methods has already been discussed — measurement of the CVP or wedge pressure. Another method is measurement of the venous oxygen saturation.

24

Oxygen saturation is a measurement
of the amount of oxygen dissolved in the
blood, and the normal value for venous blood
is greater than 60%. Ideally, this should be
done on blood taken from the CVP line or
wedge pressure catheter to insure that it is
true mixed venous blood. In a patient following myocardial infarction, a drop in oxygen
saturation between 60 and 45% means that
either shock or heart failure is present. A
drop below 45% means that both of these
pathologic processes are present.

One should not forget that there are
also certain clinical signs one can use to estimate cardiac output: urinary output, status
of sensorium and skin temperature are some
of these.

G.   PARASYMPATHETIC NERVOUS SYSTEM

Parasympathetic nervous system stimulation of the heart is represented solely by
the vagus nerves. The right vagus nerve goes
to the SA node and the left vagus to the AV
node. Vagus stimulation acts directly on the
SA node to decrease the heart rate through
pacemaker depression. It also causes a decrease in the strength of contractions of the
atria, shortening the refractory period of the
myocardium. There is a decreased rate of
conduction through the atria and Bundle of
His. This is manifested on the electrocardiogram by increased PR interval. This reflex
slowing of the heart through decreased conduction can lead to ectopic pacemaker activity and PVCs. The only beneficial effect of
vagal stimulation in times of increased cardiac output is the increased strength of myocardial contractions due to increased filling.

25

H. DECOMPENSATION

By way of review, consider what would happen if there would be a sudden decrease in circulating blood volume and venous return. This can happen in situations of hemorrhage, cardiogenic shock following myocardial infarction, severe allergic reactions, or severe infections. Sympathetic nervous system compensatory mechanisms come into play and increase the heart rate and strengthen myocardial contractions. Venoconstriction in the splanchnic bed and peripheral vessels tend to shunt blood from the peripheral to the central venous pool. Arteriolar constriction in these same areas maintains the blood pressure and vital organ perfusion. The clinical signs that all of these mechanisms are taking place are revealed by tachycardia (high pulse rate), oliguria (decreased urinary output) and cutaneous vasoconstriction manifested by cool skin with poorly dilated veins. If these compensatory mechanisms fail with further decrease in circulating blood volume, or if they do not, for some reason, develop, then shock or profound decrease in cardiac output (heart failure) results.

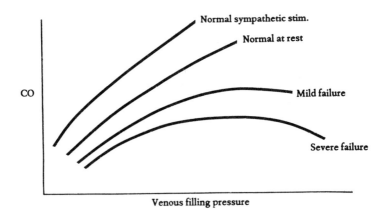

Figure 2.6   Starling Curves

26

From Figure 2.6 it can be seen that with any given diastolic filling pressure the failing heart is at a disadvantage as compared to the normal heart or the normal heart under sympathetic stimulation.

I   LEFT VENTRICULAR ACCESSMENT

For a number of years investigators have been attempting to access the functional status of the left ventricle by non-invasive techniques, that is, methods which do not require arterial or venous punctures. In the past, such methods as the Apex-Cardiogram, the Kinetocardiogram, and Balistocardiogram have been used.

Currently several methods are used to access left ventricular function. One is the Echocardiogram which makes use of pulsed high-frequency sound waves (ultrasound) to locate and plot the dimensions and movements of cardiac structures. It has also been used to determine cardiac output.

Systolic time intervals and systolic time indices are currently being used in larger centers to evaluate left ventricular function. This method requires the simultaneous recording of the phonocardiogram, the electrocardiogram, and the carotid artery pulsations. It is a fairly accurate way of determining the left ventricular status. Figure 2.7 is an illustration of the rationale upon which this method is based. The ejection time (ET) is the period of time between the opening of the semilunar valves (aortic and pulmonic) and their closure. Electromechanical systole is the period between the beginning of the q wave and the closure of the semilunar valves. The pre-ejection period (PEP) (referred to earlier in this chapter as the phase of isometric contraction) is the period from the beginning of the q wave to the closure of the semilunar valves less the ET.

From Figure 2.6 it can be seen that with any given diastolic filling pressure the resultant cardiac output is determined by the status of the heart.

27

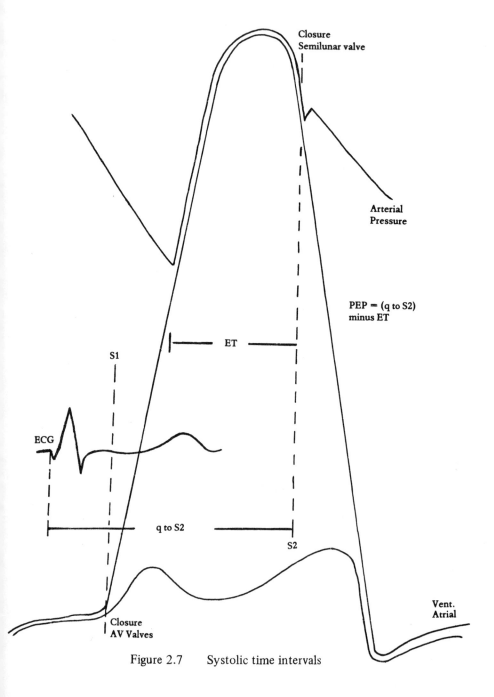

Figure 2.7   Systolic time intervals

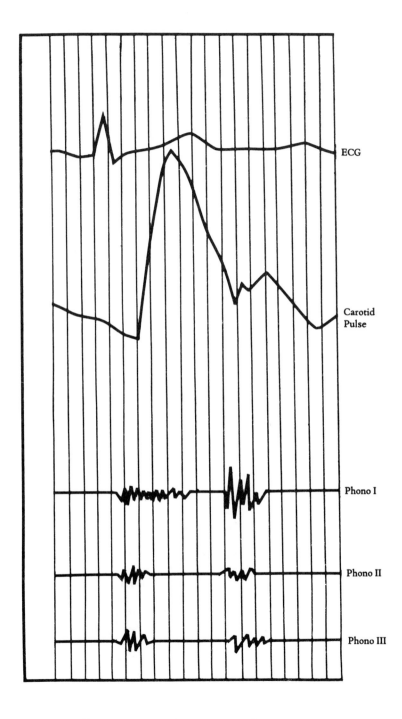

Figure 2.8   Systolic time interval tracing

The opening of the semilunar valve (in this case the aortic) is measured at the point of upsweep in the carotid pulse and the closure of the valve at the lowest inscription of the dicrotic notch. This measurement gives one the ET. A second measurement from the beginning of the q wave to the same point of the dicrotic notch gives the value for total electromechanical systole. It is a simple matter to subtract the first value (ET) from the second to get the PEP.

The significance of this measurement is that in congestive heart failure the ET is reduced at the expense of the PEP (which is increased). Both of these are reversed back to normal with digitalis.

Figure 2.8 is a typical recording used to determine these intervals.

A third method which is used to determine left ventricular function is not really a non-invasive technique since it requires a determination of the cardiac output by one of the methods mentioned earlier in this chapter. After this is done, the value obtained is divided by the surface area of the patient and the result is the Cardiac Index. This value should always be greater than 3. Any value less than 3 means heart failure.

J.   PERIPHERAL RESISTANCE

No discussion of the heart and circulation would be complete without a consideration of peripheral resistance. In essence, this is the pressure against which the heart must pump blood. When there is a high peripheral resistance (PR) the heart must work harder to pump blood from the ventricle. Less PR means less work for the heart. For practical purposes we may consider that PR is determined by the small precapillary arterioles throughout the body. These arterioles by either contracting or dilating will change the PR. When they contract the PR will rise, and when they di-

30

late (and let more blood into the capillaries) the PR will drop. These arterioles are under the control of the sympathetic nervous system and will thus be influenced by circulating catecholamines. See Chapter on Cardiac Drugs.

Peripheral resistance is of great significance in the shock state. Two types of shock have been recognized, and both may be seen in the cardiac patient. One is with peripheral vasoconstriction and high peripheral resistance. This is the classic shock situation where the natural body defenses have shunted the blood from the skin and viscera to the central circulation, and is seen in hemorrhagic and burn shock. The second type is the patient in shock with a warm dry skin and low peripheral resistance, as seen in septic shock. As already mentioned, both of these types may be seen in cardiogenic shock.

The precapillary arteriole has been called the precapillary sphincter since the caliber of these vessels determine the amount of blood that is allowed into the capillary circulation. There is another sphincter involved in the capillary circulation and this is the postcapillary sphincter. This sphincter is venules at the opposite end of the capillary bed from the arterioles and by contracting and dilating, determine the amount of blood leaving the capillary circulation. One should remember that there are quite literally miles of capillaries in the human body. Only a small percentage of these are open at any one time. If they should all open at once there would be a profound drop in the blood pressure since there simply isn't enough blood to continue circulating.

In certain circumstances (both spontaneous and iatrogenic) the postcapillary sphincters are contracted while the precapillary sphincters

31

are dilated. This allows a tremendous amount of blood into the capillary circulation which is then unavailable to the central circulation to perfuse the heart, lungs and kidneys. This is felt to be the mechanism involved in the second type of shock mentioned above. The treatment for this type of shock is to relax the postcapillary sphincter and allow the blood back into the central circulation.

The peripheral resistance may be calculated by the following formula:

$$\text{Resistance} = \frac{\text{Pressure}}{\text{Flow}}$$

or more simply:

$$\frac{\text{Peripheral}}{\text{Resistance}} = \frac{\text{Mean arterial pressure} - \text{CVP}}{\text{Cardiac output}}$$

This measurement is seldom done in clinical practice due to the need of determining the cardiac output and the mean arterial pressure, both of which require invasive techniques.

K   DISTRIBUTION OF CARDIAC OUTPUT

In the normal state the heart pumps 4.5 to 7 liters per minute. The average is about 5 liters per minute. Of this output the heart itself gets about 5% and the brain 15% (or approximately 225ml to the heart and 800ml to the brain per minute). These are obligatory amounts and are not influenced by peripheral vasoconstriction or vasodilation. The kidneys and viscera each receive 25% (or 1.5 liters) and the skin and extremities 30% (or 1.8 liters). These amounts are significantly influenced by the status of the circulation. See Figure 2.9.

32

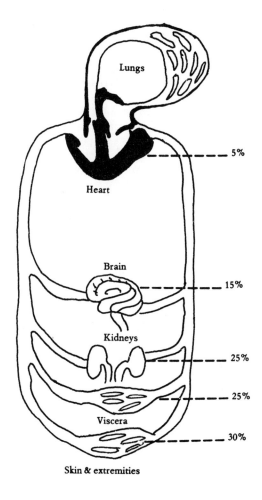

Lungs

5%

Heart

Brain

15%

Kidneys

25%

25%

Viscera

30%

Skin & extremities

4.5—7. liters/minute

Figure 2.9   Distribution of Cardiac Output

CHAPTER 3

CONDUCTION SYSTEM OF THE HEART

A.   TRANSMEMBRANE POTENTIALS

Let us now consider the remaining two
properties of cardiac tissue — automaticity
and conductivity. Automaticity is a property
of the specialized conduction system of the
heart. Conductivity is also a property of this
system and it is also a property of the muscular system — the myocardium. In order to
fully understand the nature of these two properties one has to consider the electrophysiology of the individual cardiac cell.

If one places a microscopically small
electrode on the cell membrane (the outer
surface of the cell) of a resting cell and another one inside the cell, it is found that there is
a difference in electrical potential between
the two of 90 millivolts (mV) with the outside
of the cell having a relative negative charge.
If a stimulus is then applied to the cell the
difference in electrical potential can be measured through an entire cycle and recorded on
a graph, as in Figure 3.1.

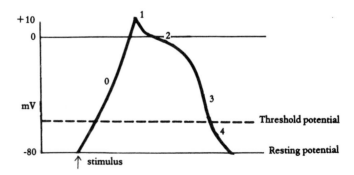

Figure 3.1   Transmembrane potential (muscle)

The baseline is called the resting potential. The critical point at which the cell will continue discharge without further stimulus is called the threshold potential and is represented by the dotted line. After the threshold potential has been reached the cell will self-propagate rapid depolarization, which is called the action potential or spike. This spike may then act as a stimulus to surrounding cells.

The transmembrane action potential is divided into five phases. O phase is the phase of rapid depolarization and is felt to be due to sodium ions entering the cell. The initial rapid repolarization (return to the resting potential) is phase 1. The slower phase of repolarization that follows is called phase 2. A return to rapid repolarization is phase 3, and final return to the resting potential is phase 4 (the diastolic period).

If a cell receives a second stimulus before full phase 4 has been reached, several responses are possible. Firstly, the stimulus may provoke no new depolarization and the cell will continue to repolarize. This period during which a new stimulus will not illicit a new response is called the absolute refractory period. Secondly, the stimulus may provoke a depolarization response which is less than maximal, or, in other words, a smaller action potential. The period during which this may happen is called the relative refractory period. Finally, the cell may fully depolarize causing a normal action potential.

There is a striking difference in phase 4 between the cells of the myocardium and the cells of the conduction system. In the myocardial cells phase 4 is a straight line and depolarization will not occur unless and until an external stimulus is applied. In the cells of the conduction system, phase 4 is characterized by slow automatic depolarization until the threshold potential is reached and then rapid depolarization ensues. This explains the automaticity of the conduction system. The action potential for a conduction system cell is represented in Figure 3.2.

35

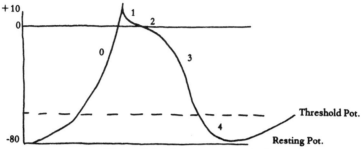
Figure 3.2   Action potential of conduction
system cell.

In the resting state the cell has a negative charge. As it depolarizes it becomes posi-
tively charged and at the same time the muscle
fiber (myofibrille) contracts. If this process
is multiplied and extrapolated to the entire
heart chamber, the result is the forceful ex-
plusion of blood from the chamber.

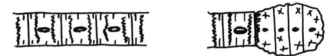
Figure 3.3   Myofibrille contraction

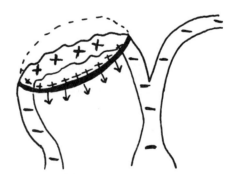
Figure 3.4   Myocardial contraction

36

Many factors influence the transmembrane potential of the conduction system cells. Phase 4 depolarization (or diastolic depolarization) is made more rapid by digitalis, catecholamines, atropine, ischemia or injury, myocardial stretch, hypokalemia, profound hypocalcemia, respiratory acidosis and hyperthermia. Phase 4 is slowed by quinidine, procainamide, lidocaine, Dilantin, Inderal, hyperkalemia, and hypothermia.

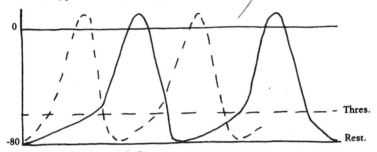

Figure 3.5   Phase 4 Influences

Changes in the threshold potential will alter the rate of discharge of the conduction cells. The threshold potential is increased by hypercalcemia and hypokalemia. It is decreased by hypocalcemia.

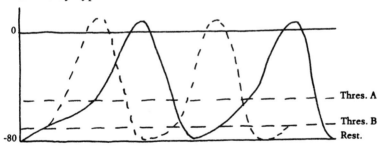

Figure 3.6   Threshold Potential Influences

The resting potential is decreased by hyperkalemia, respiratory acidosis and myocardial stretch. It is increased by hypokalemia.

37

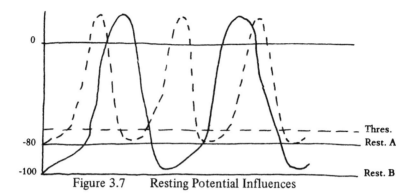

Figure 3.7   Resting Potential Influences

The effect of drugs on the transmembrane potential will be considered further in the chapter on Cardiac Drugs.

B.   CONDUCTION SYSTEM

The conduction system of the heart consists of the sinoatrial node (sinus node or SA node), the internodal pathways, the atrioventricular junction (AV node or AV junction), the Bundle of His, the right and left main bundles, the left hemibundles, and the Purkinje system. Each and every part of this system is capable of automaticity or pacemaker activity.

The SA node is the normal pacemaker of the heart. It is just a few millimeters in size and lies near the lateral junction of the atrium and superior vena cava. It also lies very near the outer surface of the heart and is therefore very vulnerable to pericarditis. However, it has been found that the pacemaking function of the SA node is relatively resistant to ischemia and nutritional needs are sparse as compared to the myocardium. It receives its blood supply from the proximal right coronary artery in 55% of cases and from the proximal left circumflex in the remaining 45%.

The SA node receives fibers from both

38

the sympathetic and parasympathetic nervous systems. The latter by way of the vagus nerve. It has been found that when the victim of an acute myocardial infarction accepts his condition as a reasonable challenge the response is mainly sympathetic (increased heart rate and blood pressure) but parasympathetic if he

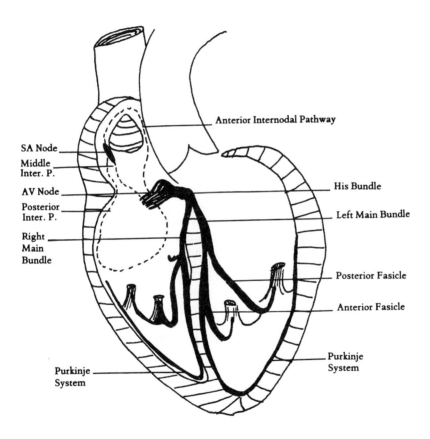

Figure 3.8   The Conduction System of the Heart

views his condition as hopeless. In the latter situation there is a strong vagotonic effect with decrease in blood pressure and profound slowing of the heart rate (bradycardia) as well as nausea and perspiration.

The SA node is also vulnerable to numerous blood-borne factors such as circulating catecholamines (epinephrine and norepinephrine), calcium, potassium, blood pH, and therapeutic drugs. These drugs will be discussed in a later chapter. The normal pacemaker rate of the SA node is approximately 80/min.

There are three pathways of conduction tissue between the SA node and the AV node. These are called internodal pathways. The middle internodal pathway goes behind the superior vena cava. It is seldom well developed and is relatively unimportant. The posterior internodal pathway takes a very long course to reach the AV node. It is probably important only as an alternate route to the AV node and as a site of ectopic rhythms. The major route is the anterior internodal pathway which takes a course through the interatrial septum to the AV node. This is also the normal route for interatrial conduction. Disruption of these pathways, as in myocardial infarction, may significantly alter normal conduction through the atria and lead to the production of arrhythmias. When acting as a pacemaker, the intrinsic rate of the pathways is 75/min.

The AV node lies deep in the interventricular septum just anterior to the opening of the coronary sinus and directly above an attachment of the tricuspid valve. It is so close to the latter that it may be affected by physical stress on the tricuspid valve as might occur with acute pulmonary hypertension. The internodal pathways all feed into the AV node. It receives its blood supply by the posterior descending branch of the right coronary artery in 90% of cases. The remaining 10% comes from the circumflex branch of the left coronary artery. This is why posterior infarctions are frequently associated with some type of heart block. Fortunately, this type of heart block usually resolves spontaneously within 72 hours. Refer to Figure 3.8.

The AV node is supplied by autonomic nerve fibers (like the SA node) and is affected by the same blood-borne influences as the SA node but in a much less significant way. The principal function of the AV node is conduction, and it is doubtful that catecholamine or calcium has any significant influence in most clinical circumstances, including myocardial infarction. Digitalis and quinidine in high doses depress AV node conduction. Acidosis has a similar effect. In low doses quinidine has an effect similar to atropine and may speed conduction through the AV node. The intrinsic pacemaker rate is 55/min.

The His Bundle takes off from the AV node and descends to the crest of the interventricular septum where it divides into a slender single right main bundle and larger left main bundle. The latter divides into several branches, the two main divisions being the anterior and posterior hemibundles, each of which goes to one of the two papillary muscles in the left ventricle.

The His Bundle and its branches consist almost exclusively of the classic Purkinje cells. It receives its blood supply mainly through the AV nodal artery (RCA), but there is also a copious collateral blood supply from various interventricular septal arteries.

If one considers the normal blood supply to the conduction system and applies

41

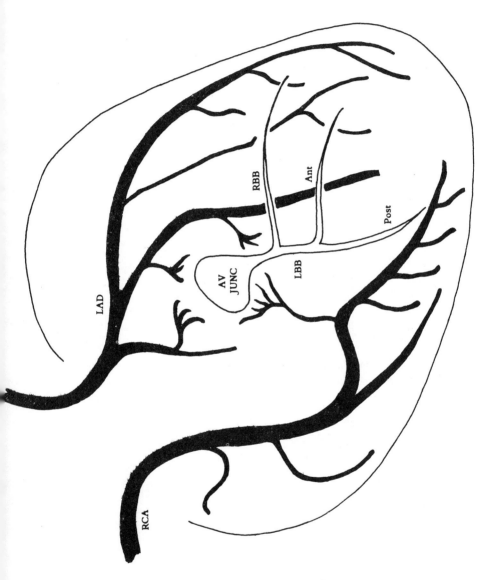

Figure 3.9 Blood Supply of the Conduction System

this knowledge to certain arrhythmias that may occur during the course of an infarction, certain prognostic indicators may be developed. For instance, a complete heart block with an anterior infarct means that all three main bundles have been damaged, and this could happen only with a very large infarct. On the other hand, the small size of the right main bundle and the comparatively small size of a lesion necessary to disrupt it, explains the much less grave prognosis of a right bundle branch block (RBBB) as compared to a left bundle branch block (LBBB).

The three main divisions of the His Bundle (right bundle, anterior and posterior branches of the left bundle) are called fasicles. A trifasicular block is one that affects all three fasicles. The blood supply to all three fasicles and two-thirds to three-quarters of the interventricular septum is by way of the anterior descending branch of the left coronary artery.

The main function of the His Bundle and its branches, like the AV node, is conduction. It is only under unusual circumstances that pacemaker activity is adopted. It should be noted here that the right main bundle has a longer refractory period than the left bundle. The intrinsic pacemaker rate is 40/min. Autonomic and blood-borne influences are the same as the AV node.

From the three main fasicles, the conduction system spreads out into a network of smaller conductive cells called the Purkinje system. The cells of the myocardium also possess the property of conductivity. As the impulse from the SA node passes through the internodal pathways, the impulse spreads to the surrounding atrial myocardium causing a contraction. Again, as the impulse passes down the His Bundle and its branches to the

43

Purkinje system, the surrounding ventricular myocardium conducts the impulse causing depolarization of the surrounding myocardial cells and contraction.

CHAPTER 4

BASIC ECG INTERPRETATION

A.   BASIC PRINCIPLES

One may translate the electrical events that take place in the conduction system of the heart during a normal cardiac cycle into a method we may observe. This method is by the underlineelectrocardiogramunderline (ECG or EKG). If a single electrode were placed on the skin and a wave of depolarization traveling toward the electrode recorded on an ECG strip, it would appear as in Figure 4.1. Note that it is recorded as a positive deflection. If the wave of depolarization were traveling away from the skin electrode, it would record a negative deflection, as in Figure 4.2.

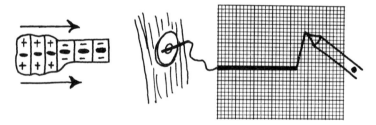

Figure 4.1   Positive Deflection on ECG

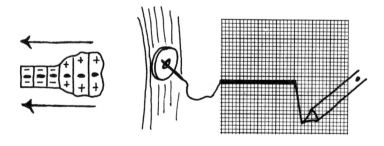

Figure 4.2   Negative Deflection on ECG

In the standard 12-lead electrocardiogram, we view the heart from 12 different vantage points. In this way, we are able to make a more accurate determination of the electrical events in the heart. The standard limb leads are placed on the right arm, left arm, and left leg. The right leg connection is the ground only. The difference in electrical potential between each of these three leads is then recorded on the ECG. Lead I describes the electrical potential difference between the right arm and the left arm, with the left arm as the positive pole. Lead II is the difference in electrical potential between the right arm and left leg, with the left leg as the positive pole. Lead III is the difference between the left arm and left leg, with the leg the positive pole.

These three leads can be thought of as a triangle (the Einthoven Triangle) and can be used to determine the electrical axis of the heart. This is of some importance when there is hypertrophy of either ventricle and in some cases of heart block. With hypertrophy of either ventricle, there will be a shift of the electrical axis to that side (to the right side with pulmonary hypertension — as in chronic lung disease; or to the left side with left ventricular hypertrophy — as in chronic hypertension.)

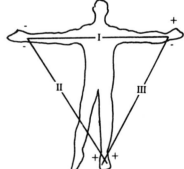

Figure 4.3   Standard Limb Leads

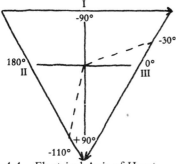

Figure 4.4   Electrical Axis of Heart

To determine the electrical axis of the heart, the forces in each standard limb lead are plotted in the triangle above and the resultant vector determined. If the electrical vector forces fall within the dotted lines, the axis is normal. Otherwise, there is abnormal axis deviation. See Figure 4.4

The following are examples of right and left axis deviations:

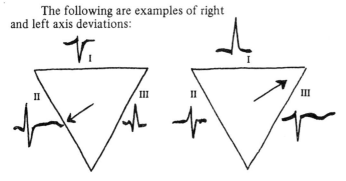

Figure 4.5   Axis Deviations

The other nine leads are the augmented limb leads (aVR, aVL and aVF) and the precordial leads. These can all be considered unipolar leads as in the examples in Figures 4.1 and 4.2. The limb leads register the electrical potential at the two arms and the left leg during a cardiac cycle, and the precordial leads measure the same electrical potential directly over the heart. These leads are useful in determining the exact site of an infarct. Precordial leads are labeled VI through V6, and their position described in Figure 4.6.

47

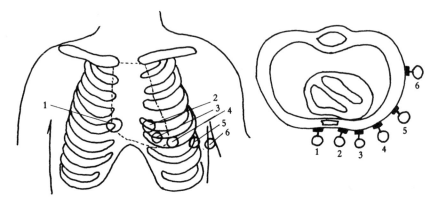

Figure 4.6   Position of Precordial Leads

The position of the leads are as follows:

VI   Right margin of the sternum at
      the 4th intercostal space.
V2   Left margin of the sternum at the
      4th intercostal space.
V3   Midway between V2 and V4.
V4   The 5th intercostal space in the
      midclavicular line.
V5   Directly lateral to V4 in the an-
      terior axillary line.
V6   Directly lateral to V4 in the mid-
      axillary line.

Other leads are occasionally used in conjunction with the precordial leads — Vr2, Vr3,
and Vr4 are placed to the right of the sternum.
V7 and V8 are placed more lateral on the left
side of the chest. Esophageal leads can also
be used.

B.   THE ELECTROCARDIOGRAM

Let us now correlate the electrical
events in the heart with the inscriptions they
make on the electrocardiogram. For illustration we will use a normal heart with the front
half cut away.

48

The pacemaker impulse originates in the SA node and spreads through the atrial myocardium. As it does so, the resultant wave of depolarization causes the upward sweep of the P wave. The P wave is the result of atrial activity and can be abnormal in those disease states which cause atrial enlargement. The P wave is always positive in Lead I, regardless of the axis.

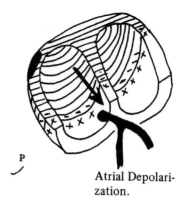

Atrial Depolarization.

There is a slight delay at the AV node (of perhaps 0.1 sec) and this accounts for the down slope of the P wave and the isoelectric part of the PR interval.

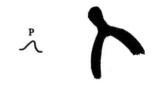

Delay at AV node

Conduction in the left main bundle is more rapid than in the right and consequently the wave of depolarization in the ventricles starts in the left side of the interventricular septum and proceeds to the right causing the first downward deflection in Leads I and II — called the q wave.

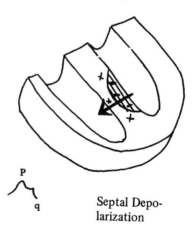

Septal Depolarization

Figure 4.7 P & q Waves

49

The wave of depolarization then spreads to the larger left ventricle and the large R wave is inscribed.

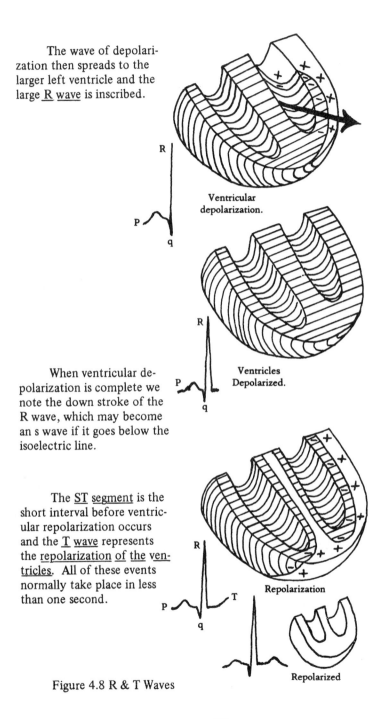

Ventricular depolarization.

Ventricles Depolarized.

When ventricular depolarization is complete we note the down stroke of the R wave, which may become an s wave if it goes below the isoelectric line.

The ST segment is the short interval before ventricular repolarization occurs and the T wave represents the repolarization of the ventricles. All of these events normally take place in less than one second.

Repolarization

Repolarized

Figure 4.8 R & T Waves

50

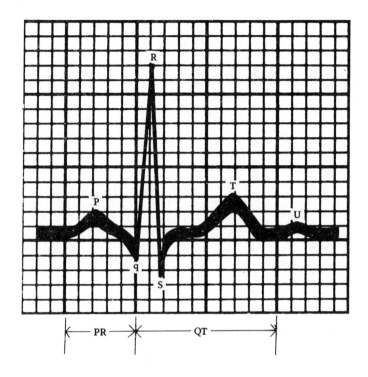

Figure 4.9   The ECG Inscriptions.

NORMAL RANGES

PR INTERVAL
    Adults   .18 to .22 seconds
    Children   .15 to .18 seconds

QRS INTERVAL   .07 to .10 seconds

QT INTERVAL	ST SEGMENT	RATE
.33−.43 sec.	.14−.16 sec.	60/min
.31−.41	.13−.15	70
.29−.38	.12−.14	80
.28−.36	.11−.13	90
.27−.35	.10−.11	100
.25−.32	.06−.07	120

Table 2.   Normal ECG Interval Values

51

The paper on which the ECG is inscribed is divided at 1 mm intervals and at 5 mm intervals. Vertically the divisions represent voltage so that each small square (1 mm) is equal to 0.1 millivolts and two large squares 1 millivolt (10 mm). The ECG machine is standardized at this relationship.

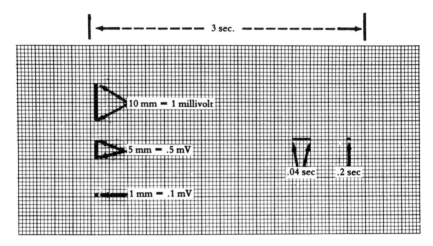

Figure 4.10   ECG Paper

The standard ECG tape is run at the speed of 25 mm/sec. This means that measuring horizontally, each small square represents .04 sec. and each large square .2 seconds. There are markings at the top of the ECG paper and the space between represents 3 seconds.

There are numerous methods by which the _heart rate_ may be calculated from the ECG, and the reader is advised to use that method which proves to be most comfortable for him. Two very simple ways of determining the heart rate are used by the author. Count the number of large squares between two consecutive R waves and divide this

52

into 300. This gives the answer in beats per minute. One can also count the number of R waves in six seconds (using the 3 second markers at the top of the ECG tape) and multiply by 10. (One can also count the number in 3 seconds and multiply by 20).

The normal time intervals for each of the electrical events inscribed on the ECG are noted in Table 2.

C. INTERPRETATION OF THE ECG

No one single test can tell us more about cardiac function than the ECG. But also, no single test can be more misinterpreted than the ECG. The clinician and nurse must always take into account the clinical picture and other laboratory data as well as the ECG before arriving at a diagnostic impression. A negative or normal ECG, especially in a suspected infarct patient or in a patient with suspected ischemic heart disease, means absolutely nothing. A change in the pattern of their ECG may mean a great deal.

When reading the ECG one should take note of a number of things. The most important are rate, rhythm, and contour of the complexes. The rate should be determined for both the atria and ventricles. Several methods have already been described for determining the ventricular rate. The atrial rate may be determined in a similar fashion, using the P waves instead of the R waves. Rhythm is often accessed by thorough examination of the P wave, and the monitor leads should be so positioned as to inscribe a distinct P wave, if possible.

1. THE P WAVE

The P wave represents depolarization of the two atria. It should be recalled that the normal pacemaker impulse arises in the SA node, high in the right atrium, and then spreads, like a ripple in water, to both atria. The P wave is always upright in Lead I, since the wave of depolarization always passes from right to left. The only exception to this is in dextrocardia, where the wave passes from left to right. The P wave is usually upright in Lead II. The average duration of the P wave is .08 seconds (two small squares) and not more than 2.5 mm in height. It is usually best seen on Lead II and precordial Lead VI.

In right atrial hypertrophy the muscle mass of the right atrium is much increased, and consequently the P wave in this condition is greater than 2.5 mm, and it is also peaked. Such a P wave is called P Pulmonale and is seen in diseases of the pulmonary vessels and with tricuspid valvular stenosis.

Hypertrophy of the left atrium results in a large muscle mass of that chamber and also a slight slowing of the wave of depolarization between the atria. This results in a double-peaked, or notched, P wave which is longer in duration than normal (greater than .12 seconds). This type of P wave is called P Mitrale and is seen in mitral valvular disease, left ventricular failure.

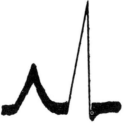 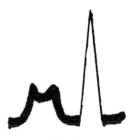

Figure 4.11 P Pulmonale;   P Mitrale

Premature atrial contractions (PACs) occur when a focus other than the SA node initiates a premature wave of depolarization in the atria. In this condition, the P wave is usually shaped differently than the normal P wave and there may be a shorter than usual PR interval. The QRS complex which follows the PAC is normal. If the P wave appears more or less normal, one can still diagnose a PAC by the interruption of the normal PP interval, and by the lack of a compensatory pause following the early QRS complex. This latter characteristic may not be present if the normal pacemaker impulse finds the atria in an absolute refractory period.

The AV node may, at times, assume pacemaker activity and cause a P wave. This may happen as a nodal or junctional premature beat or as a regular rhythm, in which case it is called a nodal or junctional rhythm. A nodal P wave may be inverted (usually in Leads II and III) or upright. It may appear before the QRS complex, in which case the PR interval is less than .12 seconds. It may also be hidden in the QRS complex or follow the QRS complex. The location of the P wave in a nodal rhythm depends on the location of the pacemaker site in the AV junction (high, middle or low).

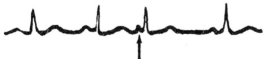

Figure 4.12 Premature Atrial Contraction

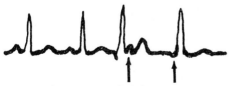

Figure 4.13 Nodal P Waves

55

An absent P wave may mean atrial fibrillation or atrial arrest (atrial asystole). A "sawtooth" pattern between the QRS complexes may mean atrial flutter. These rhythms will be discussed further in the chapter on arrhythmias.

2.   The P–R Interval

The PR interval is the period of time from the beginning of the P wave to the beginning of the q wave (or R wave, if there is no q wave). It represents conduction through the atria and AV Node. The normal PR interval varies according to the heart rate, but when over .22 seconds is diagnostic of first degree heart block. See Table 2.

3.   The QRS Complex

The QRS complex is the ventricular pattern, and describes the wave of depolarization as it passes through the ventricles. The q wave is the first downward deflection following the P wave and represents depolarization of the interventricular septum, which normally spreads from left to right. It is normally less than .04 seconds in duration and is not found in all twelve leads. It is most often seen in the right precordial leads, Lead III, and the augmented limb leads (aVR, aVL, and aVF). When seen in other leads it may mean the presence of an old infarct (scar pattern). When the q wave is wide and deep it may mean an acute infarct. See Figure 4.14.

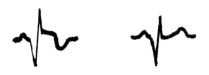

Figure 4.14   Abnormal q Waves

56

The R wave is the first positive deflection of the QRS complex (whether or not there is a preceding q wave). It represents the spread of the wave of depolarization through the rest of the ventricular muscle. In the normal heart, the R wave is very small in Lead VI and becomes progressively larger as it moves across the chest to Lead V6.

The S wave is the first negative deflection following the R wave, and may not be seen in all leads.

The normal duration of the QRS complex is no greater than .1 seconds (2½ small squares) and is unrelated to heart rate. A QRS complex of .11 seconds usually means ventricular hypertrophy and a complex of .12 seconds or longer means a bundle branch block or ventricular ectopy.

From the QRS complex one may determine the presence of left or right ventricular hypertrophy. The QRS changes are caused by the following processes: 1) Changes in the position of one ventricle in relation to the rest of the heart (as when one ventricle enlarges) will cause a change in the electrical axis of the heart. The same effect is noted with increased intracardiac pressure in any chamber of the heart. 2) Increased muscle mass in the hypertrophied ventricle will cause a shift in the electrical axis as well as an increase in the amplitude of the ventricular complexes. 3) A lessening of the distance between the heart and the chest wall will result in increased voltage of the QRS complex. 4) An increased thickness of the ventricular wall as well as some secondary changes (ischemia and fibrosis) will cause a delay in the spread of the wave of depolarization and thus a prolonged QRS complex.

57

5) Finally, because of the primary and secondary effects of hypertrophy, there will be disturbances of repolarization and consequently changes in the ST segment and T wave.

Right ventricular hypertrophy occurs as a result of increased diastolic filling (pre-load), as in atrial septal defect, pulmonic valvular insufficiency, and some rare congenital abnormalities. It can also occur as a result of systolic overloading of the ventricle (after-load) as in pulmonic valvular stenosis, or pulmonary hypertension from various causes. Right ventricular hypertrophy is diagnosed by the following criteria:

1. Right axis deviation.
2. The S wave in Lead I plus the R wave in Lead III is greater than 25 mm.
3. The ST segment in Leads II and III are depressed.
4. Evidence of either right atrial or left atrial enlargement may be present.
5. T waves in Leads II and III may be inverted.
6. The R wave in aVR is greater than 4 mm.
7. Large R wave in V1 (greater than 7 mm); S wave usually absent in V1.
8. Inverted T waves in V1 and V2.
9. The R wave is greater than the S wave in V1. The S wave is greater than the R wave in V6 in most cases.
10. A right bundle branch block pattern may be present.
11. QRS prolonged (up to .11 sec.).

See Figure 4.15.

Left ventricular hypertrophy (LVH) occurs as a result of the same two forces that
cause right ventricular hypertrophy: increased
pre-load or after-load. Diastolic overloading
can be seen in aortic insufficiency and several
congenital heart conditions. Systolic overloading is seen in aortic stenosis and arterial
hypertension. It is also noted in coronary
artery disease and in some nutritional and
metabolic diseases (Beriberi, anemia, alco-
holism, hyper and hypothyroidism).

Left ventricular hypertrophy is diagnosed
by the following criteria:
1.   The R wave in Lead 1 plus the
S wave in Lead III is greater than 25 mm.
2.   ST segment depressed in V1
and sometimes in V2.
3.   T wave flat, diphasic or inverted
in V1 and sometimes V2.
4.   Left axis deviation, usually.
5.   ST segment depressed in aVL
or aVF.
6.   Upright T wave in aVR.
7.   Voltage of the R wave in V5 or
V6 exceeds 26 mm.
8.   ST segment depressed in V4,
V5, and V6.
9.   ST segment may be elevated in
V1, V2 and V3. If this persists in all precordial leads, it may mean a ventricular aneurysm.
10.   Flat, diphasic or inverted T
waves in V4, V5 and V6.
11.   The sum of the S waves in V1
and V2 are greater than 30 mm. The sum of
the R waves in V5 and V6 are greater than
30 mm.
12.   The S wave in V2 plus the R
wave in V5 is greater than 35 mm.
13.   The R wave in V6 is taller
than in V5.
14.   Prolonged QT interval.
15.   Prolonged QRS (up to .11 sec.).

See Figure 4.16

59

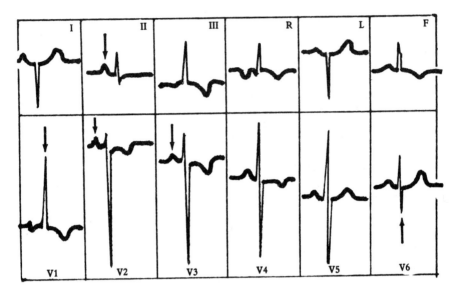

Figure 4.15   Right Ventricular Hypertrophy
(with Right Atrial Hypertrophy)

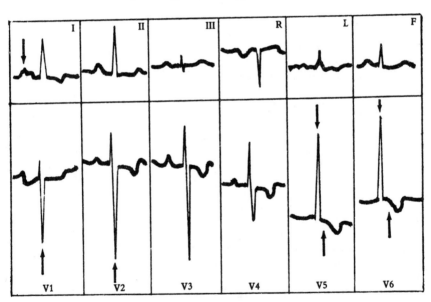

Figure 4.16   Left Ventricular Hypertrophy
(with Left Atrial Hypertrophy)

It is well to note, that seldom are all the criteria mentioned above present at the same time in either right or left ventricular hypertrophy. One must consider the clinical picture and other data before arriving at a diagnosis based on the electrocardiogram.

Ventricular ectopy is the spontaneous discharge of an ectopic focus anywhere in either ventricle resulting in a propagated wave of depolarization and ventricular contraction. It may be represented by single premature ventricular contractions (PVCs, or VPCs) or runs of two or more beats. Ventricular ectopy may also be seen as a sustained rhythm — idioventricular rhythm.

Ventricular ectopic beats (whether as a PVC or sustained rhythm) are characteristically wide (.12 seconds or longer) and bizarre. They are not preceded by a P wave, although the P wave rhythm (if present) is not disturbed by the ventricular beat. A compensatory pause usually follows the PVC before the next ventricular beat — this is because of the ventricular refractory period. The T wave is generally large and in opposite direction to the major QRS deflection and therefore usually negative (inverted). The closer the ectopic focus is to the Bundle of His the more it looks like a ventricular complex of sinus or nodal origin. See Figure 4.17.

PVCs are of great significance during the first three days following a myocardial infarction. The concept of the benign PVC versus the PVC which may herald a major arrhythmia will be discussed in a later chapter.

PVCs occur in the normal heart. They may also be associated with emotional stress, coffee, various drugs (quinidine, procainamide, atropine, digitalis, nicotine and catecholamines) and with electrolyte disturbances.

61

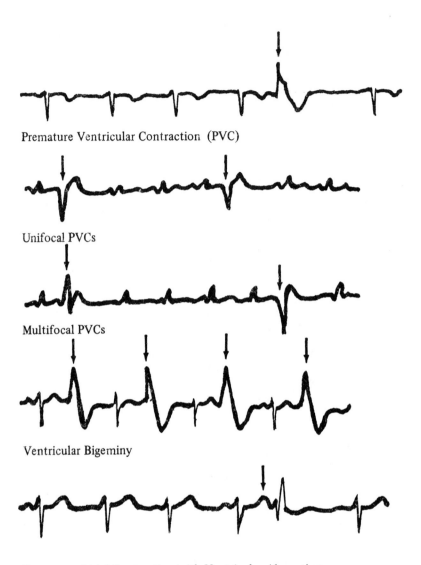

Premature Ventricular Contraction (PVC)

Unifocal PVCs

Multifocal PVCs

Ventricular Bigeminy

Premature Atrial Contraction with Ventricular Aberration

Figure 4.17 Premature Contractions.

The third major cause of prolonged
QRS complexes is bundle branch block. This
occurs when there is an interruption of conduction through any of the major branches
of the Bundle of His. This causes a widening
of the QRS to .12 seconds or more. This may
be seen in normal hearts but also in many
other circumstances such as: congenital
heart disease, rheumatic heart disease, hypertensive heart disease, several infectious diseases, excessive potassium, several drugs
(quinidine, procainamide, and digitalis),
tachycardia, coronary artery disease and myocardial infarction.

In right bundle branch block the wave
of depolarization proceeds normally down
the left main bundle and causes normal depolarization in the interventricular septum
and left ventricle. However, the wave of depolarization to the right ventricle does not
proceed by the normal channels and the
right ventricle is depolarized by conduction
through the myocardium and lesser conduction tissue. This accounts for the delay in
the complete depolarization of both ventricles and the prolonged QRS. See Figures
4.18 and 4.19.

The same is true of the left bundle
branch block, but in the opposite direction.
The ECG criteria for bundle branch block
are as follows:
      1.   QRS complex of .12 seconds
or greater.
      2.   Right bundle branch block:
Usually right axis deviation, M pattern in V1
and V2 with deep S waves in V5 and V6.
      3.   Left bundle branch block:
The QRS is slurred and notched with an M
pattern in V5 and V6. The T wave is usually
opposite in direction to the R wave in all
leads. See Figures 4.18 and 4.20.

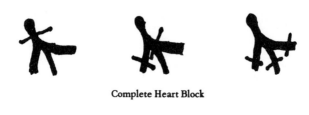

Complete Heart Block

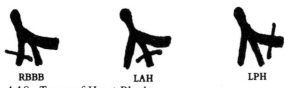

RBBB   **LAH**   **LPH**

Figure 4.18 Types of Heart Block

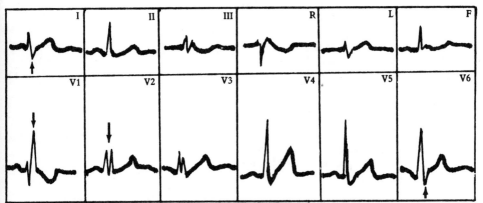

Figure 4.19 Right Bundle Branch Block

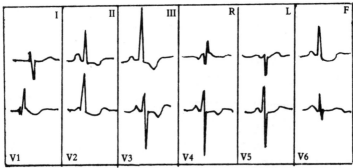

Figure 4.19a Incomplete Right Bundle Branch Block

64

Incomplete or partial bundle branch block shows the same changes in the QRS complex but less pronounced. The QRS is widened to a maximum of .11 seconds.

One may also see blocks of the two left hemibundles. In left anterior hemiblock the electrical axis is shifted markedly to the left (-60°) and the QRS complex is normal in duration or no more than .12 seconds. In left posterior hemiblock the electrical axis is to the right and there is a prolonged QRS. This latter type of block rarely occurs by itself since the left posterior hemibundle is the least vulnerable fascicle. When present, it is usually seen with right bundle branch block or left hemiblock.

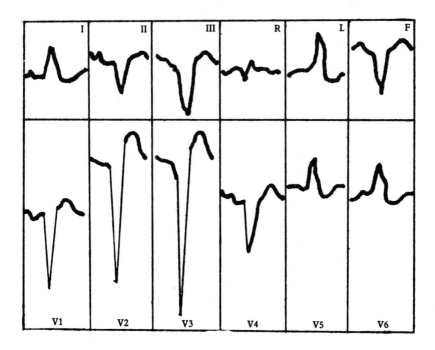

Figure 4.20 Left Bundle Branch Block

4. The ST Segment

The ST segment is the period from complete ventricular depolarization to the beginning of ventricular repolarization. Some cardiologists feel that it represents early repolarization. It is normally isoelectric, and abnormalities of the ST segment are seen as elevations or depressions of this segment. In the limb leads, elevation or depression must be greater than 1 mm to be significant. In the precordial leads, elevations must be greater than 2 mm and depressions more than 1 mm to be significant.

Elevations of the ST segment may mean infarction, pericarditis or myocardial ischemia. Depression may mean ischemia, digitalis effect, ventricular hypertrophy, or bundle branch block. The contour of ST segment is sometimes helpful in distinguishing the types of depression or elevation.

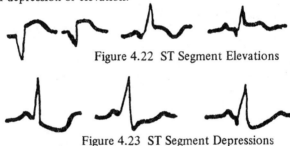

Figure 4.22 ST Segment Elevations

Figure 4.23 ST Segment Depressions

5. The T Wave

The T wave represents the final stage of ventricular repolarization. It may be abnormal in amplitude, as in infarction, myocardial ischemia, left ventricular hypertrophy, left bundle branch block and hyperkalemia (tall and peaked in the latter).

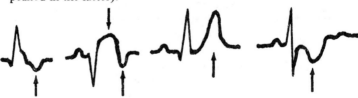

Figure 4.24 Abnormal T Waves

The T wave may also be abnormal in polarity (inverted) as in myocardial ischemia, ventricular hypertrophy, bundle branch block, pericarditis, digitalis intoxication and several metabolic abnormalities. It may also be abnormal in shape as with the broad peaked T wave in potassium intoxication.

Indeed, the abnormal T wave is so non-specific that it seldom can be used to diagnose any condition by itself.

6.   The U Wave

The U wave is occasionally seen in the ECG and is indicative of an abnormality only when it is very prominent (as in hypokalemia, hypercalcemia, digitalis and quinidine effects) or when it is negative (as with infarction, myocardial ischemia or LVH).

When present, the U wave follows the T wave by .02 to .04 seconds. It is 1 to 2 mm in height and the polarity is the same as the T wave. The U wave is caused by an after-potential, possibly of a papillary muscle.

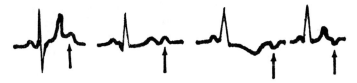

Figure 4.25 Abnormal U Waves

7.   The QT Interval

This interval is a very important measurement of ventricular function. It is measured from the onset of the q wave to the end of the T wave and represents the total time of depolarization and repolarization of the ventricles and is almost exactly equal to the ejection time. The normal QT interval shows a variation with the heart rate. See Table 2.

The QT interval is prolonged in any state causing left ventricular overload, hypocalcemia, uremia, hypokalemia, coronary artery disease, myocardial infarction, hypothermia, diabetic coma, hypertensive heart disease, rheumatic heart disease and as an effect of quinidine. The QT interval may be shortened in hypercalcemia, hyperkalemia, and as an effect of digitalis or epinephrine.

8.   The TP Interval

This is the period from the end of the T wave to the beginning of the P wave and is the period of absolute rest in the cardiac cycle — diastole. Its duration obviously depends on the heart rate. When the heart rate increases the TP interval becomes shorter.

In the past it was customary to label the small waves in the QRS complex with small letters (e.g. q wave) and the large waves with capital letters (e.g. R wave). This is no longer practiced by many cardiologists.

CHAPTER 5

ARTERIOSCLEROTIC HEART DISEASE
and
MYOCARDIAL INFARCTION

A. EXTENT OF THE PROBLEM

In this country no disease claims more
lives each year than arteriosclerotic heart disease (ASHD, coronary artery disease, ischemic heart disease). There are at least five million Americans with this disease, and between
500,000 and 700,000 deaths occur each year
from the disease or its complications. The
diagnosis is usually made in the 45 to 55 age
group, and 150,000 to 200,000 new cases
are picked up each year.

The one year mortality rate for coronary artery disease affecting one of the three
major coronary vessels is 2.5%. If two vessels
are affected the mortality rate is 10%, and if
three vessels affected the rate is 15-20%. In
patients with angina, but with unknown vessel
involvement, the mortality rate is 5-6%.

It has been variously estimated that
50-60% of patients suffering an acute myocardial infarction never reach the hospital but
succumb to sudden death due primarily to
acute arrhythmia. This is especially true of
the young patient. It is now well recognized
that a patient may suffer electrical failure
(ventricular fibrillation or complete heart
block with ventricular asystole) as a result
of an ischemic episode without true infarction. It is further believed that the ischemic
episode may be caused by spasm of a coronary
vessel and not necessarily by vessel disease.

Using the lowest estimate of mortality
from sudden death, we can assume that 50 of
100 infarct patients will reach the coronary

69

care unit (CCU). Of the 40 that survive, 30 will have an arrhythmia, 3 will go into heart failure and less than one will go into shock. Of the 10 that die after reaching the CCU, 5 will be due to arrhythmia, 3 from heart failure, and 2 from shock. See Figure 5.1.

Of all patients suffering an infarction, 50% will have had premonitory symptoms in the preceding month and 24% will have seen a physician in the preceding week. After the patient has experienced the first symptons of his infarct (chest pain, etc.) it takes between 4 and 7 hours to reach any medical aid. The psychological defense of <u>denial</u> is commonly seen. Ignorance and economic considerations are also factors which prolong the time to get to the CCU. The most influential person in getting the patient to seek medical attention is not a close family member, as one might think, but, rather, an unrelated friend or stranger. Physician delay is sometimes twice the patient delay. This is because the ECG is normal, parts of the infarction syndrome are absent, or the Friday afternoon syndrome. Administrative and triage delay after the patient reaches the hospital has long been a problem, and can account for many additional hours before the patient receives proper attention.

B.   MYOCARDIAL INFARCTION

Arteriosclerosis affects the heart in two different ways. The first way is by a progressive diminution in the caliber of the small peripheral arteries (the arterioles). This is a slow process, taking place over a period of years, and as it takes place there is a rich collateral circulation developed to meet the needs of the myocardium. In the involved vessels, there is a thickening of the <u>intima</u> (inside layer) as well as a hardening of the same layer. This results (cont'd pg 72)

70

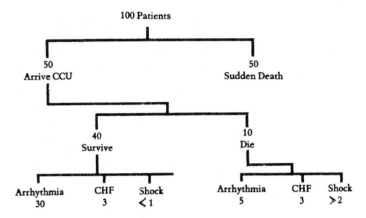

MYOCARDIAL INFARCTION

100 Patients

50 Arrive CCU	50 Sudden Death

40
Survive

10
Die

| Arrhythmia
30 | CHF
3 | Shock
< 1 | Arrhythmia
5 | CHF
3 | Shock
> 2 |

Figure 5.1   Experience in the CCU

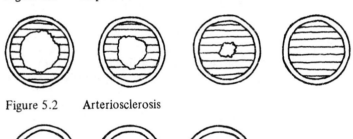

Figure 5.2   Arteriosclerosis

Figure 5.3   Atherosclerosis

(Myocardial infarction has been known
by many names: Acute MI, heart attack, coronary occlusion, coronary thrombosis, heart
stroke, heart seizure, etc. In the days before
the true pathology was understood, an infarct
was thought to be due to acute indigestion,
and one can find acute indigestion listed as the
cause of death on many old death certificates.)

71

in a decreased compliance (elasticity) of the vessel. Also, as the vessel becomes smaller in caliber, there is a decreased flow of blood through it. Figure 5.2.

This type of process can and does result in myocardial infarction, but when an infarct occurs with this type of lesion, it is usually peripheral and small.

The second way arteriosclerosis may affect the heart is by the formation of fatty deposits along the walls of the major vessels. These are called atheromatous plaques and the process of their formation is called atherosclerosis. These plaques often form in the proximal part of the major three coronary vessels (the right coronary artery, the anterior descending branch of the left coronary artery, and the circumflex branch of the left coronary artery).

If the area where the plaque is formed is occluded as with an embolus or by dislodging of the plaque itself, the resultant infarct is usually large. Figure 5.3.

Both of these types of arteriosclerosis are not exclusive to the heart and take place in many other organs. Atheromatous plaque formation is limited to larger vessels and is seen in the renal arteries and commonly in the iliac arteries.

A myocardial infarction occurs when the blood supply to a certain part of the myocardium falls below the level necessary to sustain metabolic needs. This may be due to increased demands put on the already partly occluded vessels, as seen in an infarction following a physically or emotionally stressful situation. It may also be due to the detachment of a plaque or an embolus, as seen in sudden death.

In a number of patients autopsied following sudden death, no vessel obstruction can be found. It has been presumed that these patients died of acute spasm of one of the coronary arteries, and this phenomenon of coronary spasm has been well documented by coronary arteriography.

All the possible outcomes following an acute myocardial infarction along with the complications are noted in Figure 5.4. The patient may experience primary ventricular arrhythmia (fibrillation) and die immediately. On the other hand, he may experience infarction, have no complications, and enjoy an uneventful recovery. Between these two extremes, all sorts of difficulties may arise, including congestive heart failure, shock, and secondary arrhythmia.

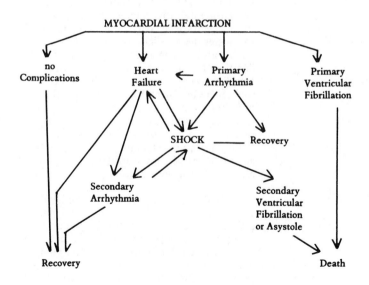

Figure 5.4   Possible Outcomes of Acute MI

Two factors must be taken into consideration in accessing the significance of a myocardial infarction — site and size. They are of equal importance. A small occlusion of the AV nodal artery which will infarct the AV node and Bundle of His may be a more life-threatening lesion than a much larger infarct affecting one-third of the left ventricular myocardium.

Occlusion of the anterior descending branch of the left coronary artery accounts for approximately 70% of major infarcts. The right coronary artery accounts for another 30%, and the circumflex for 10-15%. Occlusion of the left main coronary trunk is very rare.

The size of an infarction is determined by: 1) the extent of the occluded blood supply; 2) the amount of collateral circulation; and 3) the oxygen demands of the myocardium. There are certain conditions which, by increasing the oxygen demands of the injured or ischemic myocardium, can cause the infarct to enlarge. Positive inotropic agents, especially isoproterenol and to a lesser degree digitalis, will do this. Tachycardia, by increasing the work of the heart, and acidosis, by interfering with intracellular enzyme systems, will also do this. Increased stretch of myocardial fibers, as in hypertension (increased afterload) or an enlarged heart, as in failure (increased preload) also increase oxygen demands of the myocardium. An infarct causing damage to 40% of the myocardium will almost assuredly result in death.

Several factors can improve or limit the size of the infarction. Hypertonic glucose is one of these. Controlling hypertension (to 120 mm Hg systolic) is another. In shock, a counterpulsating balloon pump will help limit the size of the infarct by improving perfusion of the coronary arteries.

C.   DIAGNOSIS OF MYOCARDIAL INFARCTION

The clinician relies on four sources of
information to make the diagnosis of acute
myocardial infarction. The first and most useful source of information is the history. The
chest pain a patient describes with an acute
myocardial infarction is usually that of in-
tense pressure in the precordium (the chest
overlying the heart) ("a weight is sitting on
my chest"), and is often described by a gripped
fist held over the heart. The pain may radiate
to the left shoulder and down the left arm or
to the jaw. In some patients, the pain has
been described as "sharp". In others, the
pain may radiate to the right arm. The common factor is the pain in the precordial area,
which may or may not be of the pressure-type
and may or may not radiate to either arm or
jaw. The pain is often associated with short-
ness of breath (dyspnea), nausea (and sometimes vomiting), and sweating (diaphoresis).
Fainting (syncope) may occur.

If the above occurs in a patient with a
history of heart disease or angina, diabetes
mellitus, hypertension, obesity, or a strong
family history of ASHD, one is rather safe in
making a presumptive diagnosis of acute myocardial infarction. We will consider Risk
Factors in a later chapter.

The second source of information to
diagnose myocardial infarction is the physical
examination. Here the presence of a gallop
rhythm is most significant. The atrial gallop
rhythm is more common, but the ventricular
diastolic gallop is also rather frequent. The
latter can mean early cardiac decompensation
and may be the earliest indication for treatment of pump failure. In both instances, the
louder the gallop the poorer the prognosis.
Both of these rhythms are best heard using
the bell stethoscope with the patient in the
left lateral recumbent position. The presence

75

of any gallop rhythm should alert the clinician to underlying heart disease or to im-
pending myocardial infarction.

The third source of information concerning infarction comes from the electrocardiogram. To understand the ECG changes
that one looks for in myocardial infarction
it must be understood that in the area of infarction the myocardial cells are dead and
cannot be either depolarized or repolarized.
This amounts to an electrical inert area and
its size, of course, depends on the size of the
infarct. In the normal left ventricle, the sum
of the electrical forces from deploarization
of the ventricle is directed toward the left
foot, and is represented by the large arrow in
Figure 5.5. This is recorded in Leads II and
III as a positive deflection. If a portion of
the myocardium becomes electrically inert,
as with an infarction, the sum of the electrical forces will be changed, as in Figure
5.6. The result is the formation of a wide
q wave in Leads II and III (in an inferior infarction).

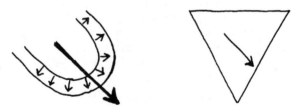

Figure 5.5   Normal Left Ventricular Vector

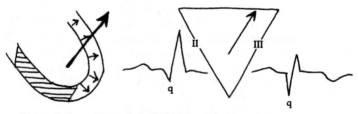

Figure 5.6   Ventricular Vector of Acute MI

76

An electrode placed directly over the infarcted area will record the wave of depolarization of the opposite side of the heart, and this has been described as a "window" in the heart. In Figure 5.7 one may note the typical electrocardiographic changes of a large subepicardial infarct. The earliest ECG sign of an infarct is ST elevation. This is followed by a q wave and by T wave inversion. The pathologic q wave is the hallmark of an acute MI. This q wave is .04 seconds or more and appears in leads that do not normally show a q wave.

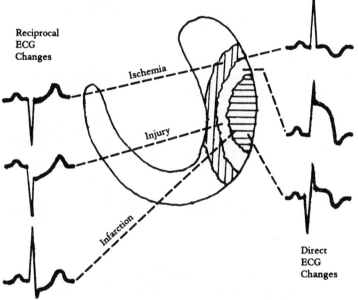

Reciprocal ECG Changes

Ischemia

Injury

Infarction

Direct ECG Changes

Figure 5.7　　ECG Changes in Acute MI

In the zone of actual infarction, called the necrotic zone, we find the deep q wave, an elevated ST segment and an inverted T wave. In the zone of injury (the injured but not dead area immediately surrounding the infarct) we do not see the q wave but do see the elevated ST segment and inverted T wave. In the zone of ischemia (just outside the zone

77

of injury) the q wave and ST elevation are absent but, the inverted T wave is present. Reciprocal changes are noted 180° from the infarct.

As the infarct evolves the ST segment slowly returns to the baseline and the T wave becomes upright. The pathological q wave may disappear but also may remain along with the inverted T wave to produce a scar pattern. See Figure 5.8.

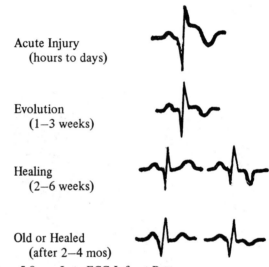

Acute Injury
(hours to days)

Evolution
(1–3 weeks)

Healing
(2–6 weeks)

Old or Healed
(after 2–4 mos)

Figure 5.8   Late ECG Infarct Patterns

The above discussion has been concerned with the classical changes in a fairly large subepicardial infarction. However, an infarct may occur at various sites in the heart, and the diagnosis is not always so clear-cut. Infarcts may occur subendocardial, subepicardial, intramural (entirely within the myocardium) or transmural (involving the entire thickness of the myocardium). Small infarcts of any variety may not produce the classic signs noted above. In about 40% of all infarcts the classic signs will not appear.

If the diagnostic pattern is not present in a suspected infarct patient, serial electrocardiograms are often quite useful. The diagnostic pattern may appear later or other ECG changes may evolve to make the diagnosis. In the smaller infarct noted above, one may only see ST segment elevation, or perhaps a transient q wave or T wave inversion. Serial electrocardiograms are always of significance even in those cases where the diagnosis is firmly established. In this way, one can follow the evolution or extension of an infarct. ONE CAN NEVER EXCLUDE THE DIAGNOSIS OF AN INFARCTION BY THE ELECTROCARDIOGRAM.

The significance of the location of an infarction has already been discussed (page 74). We may divide all infarcts into either anterior or posterior — depending on which aspect of the heart is involved. Anterior infarcts are usually due to occlusion of the anterior descending branch of the left coronary artery but may also be due to occlusion of proximal branches of the circumflex. Posterior infarcts are due to occlusion of the right coronary artery and rarely to occlusion of distal branches of the circumflex. The more common types of infarcts along with their characteristic ECG pattern is shown in Figures 5.9 and 5.10.

The fourth and last source of information to make a diagnosis of acute infarction comes from the serum enzymes. When a cell dies or is damaged, part of the intracellular contents find their way into the general circulation and can be measured in the laboratory. Myocardial cells are rich in certain enzymes. Among these are glutamic oxalacetic transaminase (SGOT), lactic dehydrogenase (LDH), and creatine phosphokinase (CPK). These enzymes are released from the damaged cell at different rates and their corresponding rate of rise in the serum following an acute myocardial infarction is different. See Figure 5.11. This is further complicated by the fact

79

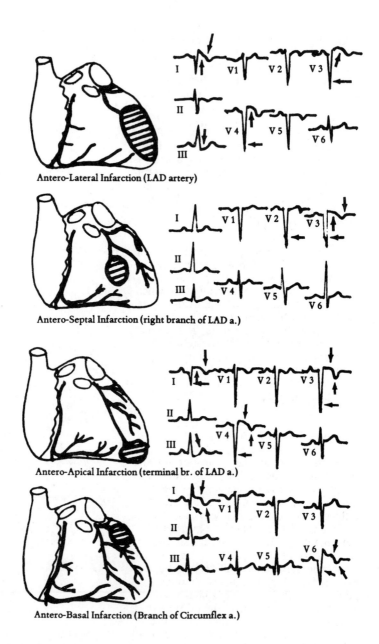

Antero-Lateral Infarction (LAD artery)

Antero-Septal Infarction (right branch of LAD a.)

Antero-Apical Infarction (terminal br. of LAD a.)

Antero-Basal Infarction (Branch of Circumflex a.)

Antero-Basal Infarction (Branch of Circumflex a.)
Figure 5.9 Anterior Infarctions

80

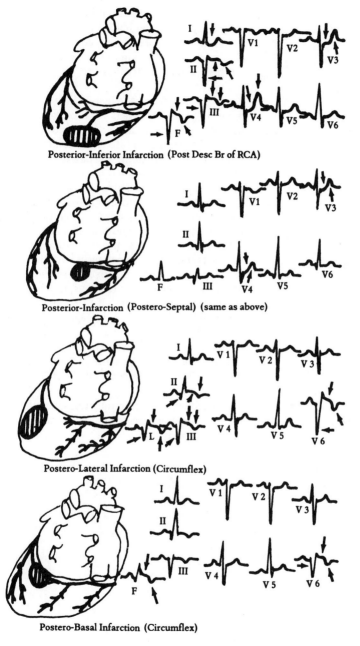

Posterior-Inferior Infarction (Post Desc Br of RCA)

Posterior-Infarction (Postero-Septal) (same as above)

Postero-Lateral Infarction (Circumflex)

Postero-Basal Infarction (Circumflex)

Figure 5.10 Posterior Infarctions.

81

that no enzyme has yet been found which is exclusively in myocardial cells. There are a number of other diseases and conditions which can cause a rise in the serum enzymes which we can currently measure.

Of some diagnostic help,is the fact that two of the above enzymes can be separated into various fractions in some laboratories — LHD can be separated into five fractions and CPK into three fractions. Certain of these fractions are found more often in cardiac muscle than in other tissues. For instance, LDH fraction II is normally greater than fraction I. Following a myocardial infarction, fraction I becomes greater than fraction II, and when the relationship returns to normal we can assume that the patient is over the critical period. If the crossover to the normal ratio has not occured by ten days, it is a very poor prognostic sign. If CPK fraction II is found in the serum, it is diagnostic of acute myocardial infarction. If none is found, an infarct cannot be excluded. Intramuscular injections during the acute stage of an infarction make CPK determinations useless.

Daily enzyme determinations can often be of great help in deciding whether an infarct has occurred.

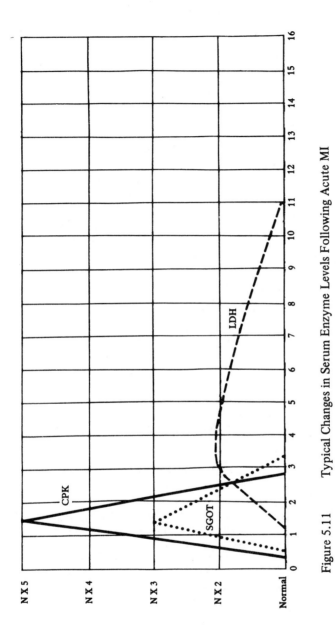

Figure 5.11   Typical Changes in Serum Enzyme Levels Following Acute MI

83

CHAPTER 6

ARRHYTHMIAS

A.   CLASSIFICATION

Cardiac arrhythmias occur at some time in 90% of all acutely infarcted patients and is the most common complication of acute myocardial infarction. During the past decade, more papers have been written and more research done on this subject than on any other phase of acute coronary care. Consequently, we have come to recognize that a vigorous attack on the arrhythmia can do more to prevent a fatal outcome following an acute MI than any other approach. The aims of therapy of arrhythmias are to prevent the progression to a more serious arrhythmia and to improve cardiac output.

One can study cardiac arrhythmias according to various classifications. Some classify them according to their rate. In most standard textbooks, they are classified according to their origin (atrial, junctional or ventricular), which has much merit for the cardiologist. One of these we can recommend as an essential part of every CCU. This is the book by Samuel Bellet, <u>Essentials of Cardiac Arrhythmias</u>, 1972, Saunders. In everyday clinical practice and in teaching acute coronary care it is useful to divide the arrhythmias into three groups according to their clinical significance: 1) arrhythmias of electrical instability, 2) bradyarrhythmias, and 3) arrhythmias of pump failure.

B.   ARRHYTHMIAS OF ELECTRICAL INSTABILITY

The most common type of arrhythmia following an acute myocardial infarction is the ventricular ectopic beat or premature ventricular contraction (PVC or VPC). This is also the most important arrhythmia because it can lead to ventricular fibrillation. It occurs in 80% of MIs and is due to a lowered threshold during the vulnerable period in the area of the infarct, as well as the injured and ischemic areas. The cause may be hypoxia, increased circulating catecholamines, increased stretch on the myocardial fibers, or local hyperkalemia. In any case, the transmembrane potential of the affected cells shows an increased slope of slow depolarization. This amounts to enhanced automicity and one also sees re-entry activity.

Nearly 90% of PVCs originate in the left ventricle and are due to ASHD of one degree or another. Only 10% originate in the right ventricle and are not due to ASHD. PVCs can be either benign or malignant. The latter are seen in pairs or runs, occur on the T wave or show a multifocal origin. In practice, if a PVC is seen more often than five times per minute, it should be considered malignant and treated accordingly.

The electrocardiographic characteristics of the PVC have been discussed in an earlier chapter (see page 61).

Ventricular tachycardia occurs in 28% of infarct patients and has the same ominous prognosis as the malignant PVC. In ventricular tachycardia (VT) the QRS complexes are wide (.12 seconds or greater) and usually bizarre – they resemble PVCs. The rate is 210 or less. There is usually A-V dissociation, although one occasionally sees retrograde conduction (i.e. the atria contract in response to a wave of depolarization coming up from an irritable focus in the ventricle). One should be able to see captured beats and fusion beats. Captured beats are an occasional normal QRS complex preceded by a P wave. This occurs when the depolarizing impulse from the SA node arrives at the AV node at just the right time to be transmitted down the ventricular conduction system to set off a normal contraction. A fusion beat is seen as a QRS complex midway in contour and size between the wide and bizarre ventricular complex and the normal QRS complex. This occurs when there is simultaneous depolarization from the SA node and the irritable focus in the ventricle. See Figures 6.2 and 6.3.

With any ventricular rhythm (VT included), if fusion beats or capture beats are not seen, one must conclude there is complete A-V block, and certain precautions must be taken before treatment is instituted. In complete A-V block, the atria and ventricles are contracting in a completely independent way. Sinus impulses are not transmitted past the AV node, and idioventricular impulses are not transmitted retrograde to the atria. If the ectopic ventricular focus is abolished in this situation, there will be no mechanism to initiate ventricular contraction, and the result is ventricular asystole.

There are several conditions seen on the ECG which may confuse the diagnosis of PVCs. The PVC is often confused with the PAC with aberrant conduction. This latter phenomenon usually looks like a RBBB complex in lead V1. Look for the P wave and absent compensatory pause. The general appearance of these conplexes is seen in Figure 6.4.

86

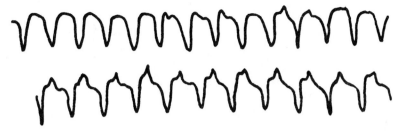

Figure 6.1   Ventricular Tachycardia.

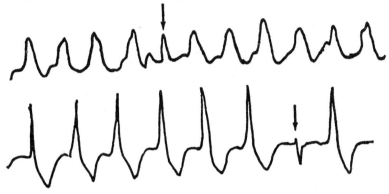

Figure 6.2   Ventricular Tachycardia with
              Capture Beats.

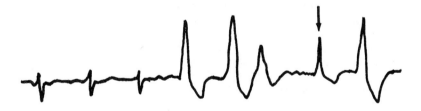

Figure 6.3   Ventricular Tachycardia with
              Fusion Beat.

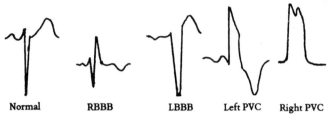

Normal   **RBBB**   **LBBB**   Left PVC   Right PVC

Figure 6.4   QRS Complexes

Parasystole may also be confused with PVCs, and there is one type of PVC that does not show a compensatory pause — the interpolated PVC. Parasystole is usually due to digitalis.

Ventricular tachycardia may be confused with a rate dependent bundle branch block. Some BBBs occur only with tachycardia. This is especially true with RBBB. About 90% of tachycardias with an apparant RBBB are not VT.

1.   Treatment

The aim of treatment for PVCs or VT is to prevent ventricular fibrillation (VF). If treatment is performed in a vigorous and expeditious way, the incidence of ventricular fibrillation in the CCU can almost be abolished.

The current accepted treatment for the malignant type of PVC is an immediate bolus of Lidocaine of 50 to 100 mg followed by the continuous intravenous infusion of Lidocaine at the rate of 1 mg per minute (15 drops per minute by microdrip) and slowly increased up to 4 mg per minute (60 drops per minute by microdrip) if necessary to keep the PVCs less than five per minute. This may seem rather radical treatment for what appears to be a rather innocuous event. The patient appears well, his vital signs are stable, but we see numerous multifocal PVCs on the monitor. We now know from very sound experience that the malignant PVC may lead to ventricular

88

tachycardia and then ventricular fibrillation. Even if cardioversion for VF is successful, two-thirds of those patients cardioverted for VF will die within five hours.

Follow-up therapy for PVCs, after the intravenous Lidocaine, is oral procainamide or propranolol, and finally diphenylhydantoin if the others are unsuccessful. If all the oral preparations are unsuccessful, the ultimate resource is the pacemaker to "override" the ectopic focus and limit the number of PVCs.

The therapy for ventricular tachycardia is essentially the same as for PVCs, except that if Lidocaine (in the same doses) is not successful, one goes immediately to DC cardioversion. Cardioversion (countershock) is felt to work in this type of arrhythmia because of its ability to depolarize the entire ventricle at the same time and thereby bring all the tissue into the same phase for subsequent organized electric activity.

However, one should never cardiovert a rhythm with complete heart block — such as VT — without capture or fusion beats. The reason for this is noted above. The one exception is when a pacemaker (either transvenous or indwelling) is in place and ready to function on demand. With a pacemaker in place, one may cardiovert and if a regular rhythm does not result, the pacemaker can be turned on immediately.

The prognosis for the above two arrhythmias is good if immediate therapy is instituted to prevent the common complication of ventricular fibrillation. If VF does occur, there is only one treatment and that is by DC cardioversion at the maximal setting on the defibrillator. If immediate conversion to a regular rhythm is not obtained, counter-

89

shock must be repeated and advanced life support measures begun (such as Lidocaine bolus and drip, bicarbonate, epinephrine, and IV and CPR). Ventricular fibrillation is due to an abnormal buildup of metabolites or potassium in the ischemic tissue and not due to hypoxia (as was once felt to be the case).

There are several theories to explain the occurrence of ventricular ectopy. The re-entry mechanism is postulated to explain PVCs with a fixed coupling interval and other arrhythmias. By this theory, if there is an area in the myocardium with a depressed excitability, the surrounding myocardium will depolarize first, and then when the depressed area finally depolarizes, it will initiate a wave of depolarization which will be propagated to the surrounding tissue. The circus movement theory postulates a continuous movement of ectopic excitation occurring in a circular fashion in the myocardium of conductive tissue. Both of these theories have validity and may be used to explain several different types of ectopy. See Chapter 9 for a further discussion of this topic.

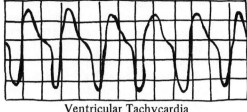

Ventricular Tachycardia

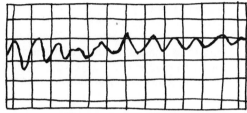

Ventricular Fibrillation

Figure 6.5   Ventricular Arrhythmias

C.   BRADYARRHYTHMIAS

Bradyarrhythmias are defined by a heart rate below 60 and occur in about 25% of infarct patients and usually in small infarcts. The most common type is sinus bradycardia. This is a result of a strong vagotonic reflex (see page 25) and occurs in 44% of posterior-inferior infarcts. Although this rhythm usually occurs with small infarcts, the bradycardia itself may be potentially dangerous. The slow heart rate enhances electrical instability and may lead to escape PVCs or VT and reduces the threshold for VF.

A marked bradycardic response has been demonstrated in all diving land vertebrates. This is due to an oxygen conserving mechanism which lowers the heart rate and thereby in-creases the stroke volume. The blood pressure rises as the peripheral resistance increases to shunt the blood from the skin and viscera.

91

Anaerobic metabolism eventually intervenes with a rise in serum lactate and potassium and a decrease in pH. This entire response can be initiated by a deep feeling of fear with an inappropriately strong vagal response, especially when mixed with a feeling of despair or hopelessness. Vagomimetic drugs, such as morphine sulfate, enhance this response.

Weiss demonstrated 35 years ago that sudden death may occur under severe emotional stress in the presence of ASHD. This may account for the efficacy of Voodoo curses. In summary, sudden death may occur due to an exaggerated bradycardic response, when combined with fear, hopelessness or pain.

In addition to the above mechanisms, other factors may enhance the occurrence of sinus bradycardia. Dilatation of the sinus node artery, increased potassium from ischemic or necrotic tissue, changes in the blood pH, reduced secretion of catecholamines may all contribute to bradycardia.

In the normal heart, cardiac output depends on heart rate and stroke volume. If one is lowered, the other compensates to maintain the cardiac output. However, in the infarcted heart where there is left ventricular dysfunction, a decreased heart rate cannot be compensated for by an increased stroke volume. The result is a decreased cardiac output, anaerobic metabolism, and decreased perfusion of the heart, brain and kidneys. In addition, the left ventricular filling pressure may rise to the point that pulmonary congestion and edema may occur. This is all due to inappropriate bradycardia.

There is another side to this coin. Epstein has shown that bradycardia exerts a protective influence on the heart in dogs, and that atropine predisposes them to the development of arrhythmias. Data from patients does not support the contention that uncomplicated bradycardia is associated with increased mortality. On the contrary, there seems to be a diminished risk in these patients. This applies when there is no sign of pump failure, such as hypotension. There is also the possibility that the positive chronotropic effect of atropine may cause an extension of the infarct, as does isoproterenol by its similar effect on the heart rate. The conclusion that can be drawn concerning vagal stimulation during ischemia is that it diminishes ventricular vulnerability to fibrillation.

Junctional (nodal) rhythms are often of the bradycardia type. The intrinsic rate of the AV node is 55/min. The P wave is always positive in AVR and the PR interval is usually shorter than normal. The P wave is usually negative in those leads in which it is usually positive. In 80% of cases with a junctional rhythm, the P wave precedes the R wave, but it may also occur after the QRS and may even be buried in the QRS.

The current treatment for the above bradycardias depends on the patient's condition. The patient with bradycardia in the first few hours following an infarct may appear to be in frank shock. Elevation of the feet and IV atropine may rapidly reverse the situation. If the patient shows no sign of pump failure or electrical instability, no treatment is indicated. If pump failure or PVCs are present the treatment is with a bolus of .6 to 1.0 mg of atropine given IV. If this is unsuccessful, a pacemaker should be used.

PVCs resulting from a bradycardia are called escape beats. They are usually benign.

The prognosis for the above arrhythmias is excellent with appropriate therapy when indicated. Complications of a sustained treatable bradycardia of the above type is asystole or ventricular fibrillation.

Heart block is another type of bradycardia which must be considered. Heart block occurs in three degrees of severity. A first degree heart block is a delay in conduction from the SA node to the AV node. It occurs in 7–10% of infarcts, and is represented on the ECG by a prolonged PR interval. No therapy is indicated by a first degree heart block.

A second degree heart block can be one of two types, and occurs in 5% of posterior inferior infarcts, and is usually transient. The first type is the Mobitz Type I (which is the same thing as the Wenckebach Phenomenon) and is a progressive prolongation of the PR interval until there is a dropped ventricular beat. This is the most common of the second degree blocks.

A Mobitz Type II block is the less common of the two types of second degree block, and is the dropping of a ventricular beat without previous prolongation of the PR interval. In its more advanced forms, there may be several atrial contractions which are not transmitted and may result in long periods of ventricular asystole. These periods are usually intermittent and must be distinguished from sinus arrest and other conditions which may give rise to the same phenomenon. Like the third degree heart block, which we will consider below, the Mobitz Type II is usually due to a large anterior infarct and may be permanent.

See Figures 6.6, 6.7, and 6.8.

94

Third degree heart block (complete heart block) is when the atria and ventricles are contracting in response to an entirely different pacemaker. The atria usually respond to the normal SA node at the rate of 70÷80/minute, while the ventricles respond to an ectopic pacemaker in the AV node, Bundle of His, or upper part of the main bundles at a rate of 20—40/minute. While the SA node and atria may respond to autonomic influences, the ventricles usually show little effect of this stimulation, and periods of ventricular asystole may occur.

Complete heart block (like the other ventricular bradycardias) can lead to PVCs and VT and/or VF, and is therefore a rather dangerous situation. When it occurs with an inferior infarct there is a low mortality because the conduction system is not usually seriously injured. When it occurs with an anterior infarct and complete bundle branch block, there is a high mortality due to the wide extent of an infarct necessary to produce such an event. See Figures 6.9 and 6.9a.

The only currently accepted treatment for Mobitz Type II and third degree heart block is the insertion of a demand pacemaker. In the acute MI patient this is usually the transvenous type. No drugs have any beneficial influence on these more advanced blocks and may even be detrimental.

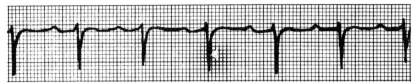

Figure 6.6   First Degree AV Block

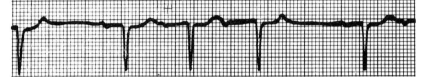

Figure 6.7   Second Degree AV Block (Mobitz 1)

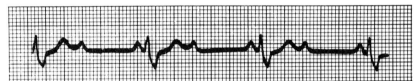

Figure 6.8   Second Degree AV Block (Mobitz II)

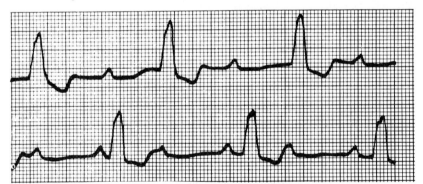

Figure 6.9   Complete Heart Block with Idio-
Ventricular Rhythm

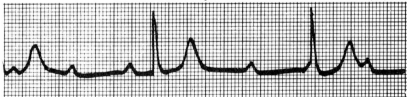

Figure 6.9a Complete Heart Block with Idio-Nodal Rhythm

D. ARRHYTHMIAS OF PUMP FAILURE

These arrhythmias occur in 20% of myocardial infarctions and are supraventricular in origin. They are associated with a poor prognosis. They occur most especially with left ventricular failure and 75% occur with anterior infarcts. These arrhythmias are usually of the tachycardia type.

Sinus tachycardia occurs in 35% of infarctions and is defined as a sinus rate of 100–150/minute. It is diagnosed by determining the heart rate and finding a P wave preceding each QRS complex on the ECG. The proper PR interval should also be present. A sustained tachycardia must be treated, and the drug of choice following a recent infarction is a rapid-acting digitalis glycoside; such as digoxin, deslanoside, or quabain. One should first be sure that the tachycardia is not due to sympathetic stimulation (as with catecholamine drugs), but rather to heart failure, which is the usual cause of a sustained tachcardia.

Atrial flutter is a regular atrial rate of 250–350/minute. The ventricular response is variable and may be 1:1, 1:2, 1:3, 1:4, etc. The immediate treatment is with digitalis to increase the AV block and reduce the ventricular rate to 100 or less. The eventual treatment is cardioversion followed by digitalis and quinidine. The diagnosis is made by the ECG by finding F waves (or flutter waves). These waves give a "sawtooth" appearance to the isoelectric line. See Figure 6.10.

97

Atrial fibrillation is a very common arrhythmia and may be present in many patients before they have an infarct. The atrial rate is difficult to count, but is between 350–600/minute. The ventricular rate is variable, but in many cases is also very rapid. The first approach to treatment is to reduce the ventricular rate to a functional level by increasing the AV block. This is done with digitalis in doses large enough to reduce the ventricular rate — often very large doses. A second approach is with propranolol. Quinidine and cardioversion are also used if conversion to a sinus rhythm is felt to be necessary. Diagnosis is made by the electrocardiogram. The ventricular rate is usually somewhat irregular and there are no discernable P waves, although the QRS complexes are normal in width and contour (thus excluding an idioventricular rhythm). The isoelectric line is often flat, but may be somewhat jagged. See Figure 6.11.

In order to complete the discussion of supraventricular tachycardias, atrial tachycardia must be considered. This is a rate of 150–250/minute usually with a 1:1 ventricular response. This may or may not be associated with heart disease and is seldom seen following an acute infarction. The onset of this arrhythmia is usually abrupt and for that reason is often referred to as paroxysmal atrial tachycardia (PAT). It may last only a few minutes, but also may last for weeks. These episodes of PAT are of little consequence as far as cardiac function is concerned, but are often very disturbing to the patient. Diagnosis is made from the history of abrupt onset and the ECG finding of a tachycardia with P waves that are not quite normal (although, in many cases, they may be indistinguishable from the normal P wave).

The first mode of treatment is by vagal stimulation (carotid sinus pressure or eyeball pressure) and this usually interrupts an attack. The ultimate treatment is by digitalis, but many other drugs may be tried first, such as quinidine or aspirin (which oddly enough, has been implicated as the cause of PAT). The author has found phenobarbital to be quite useful in this condition and one is reminded that emotional stress may be one of the causative factors of PAT. Propranolol has also been very successful in treating this condition.

Nodal tachycardia is a rather rare condition and is treated the same as the arrhythmias noted above. Suspect Digitalis toxicity.

Premature atrial contractions (atrial extrasystoles, PACs) are a fairly common arrhythmia following an acute MI and if associated with aberrant conduction may mask as a PVC. Their occurrence is rather nonspecific and may be associated with many diseases and conditions and may also be seen in normal hearts. When occurring during the course of an infarction they may mean a pulmonary embolus or various drug effects. Hypokalemia may also be a cause. Diagnosis is made by the ECG. The P wave is premature, is different from the normal P wave and may be inverted. The preceding T wave may be distorted by the premature P wave. The QRS complex is usually normal except when the ectopic excitation occurs during the refractory period of the ventricular cycle. The result is aberrant conduction and "pseudo" —PVCs. The aim of treatment is to prevent the emergence of atrial flutter or fibrillation and this is done with digitalis, quinidine or inderal. See Figure 6.12.

99

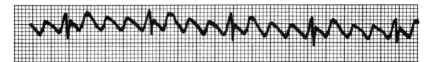

4:1   AV Conduction.

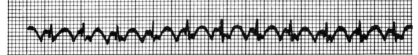

2:1   AV Conduction

Figure 6.10   Atrial Flutter

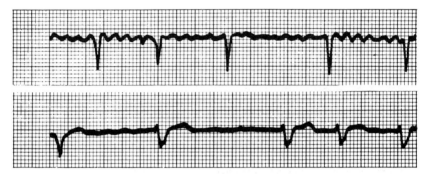

Figure 6.11   Atrial Fibrillation.

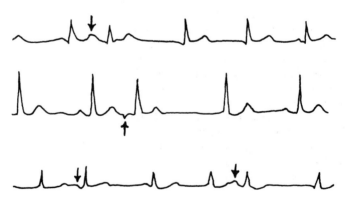

Figure 6.12   Premature Atrial Contractions.

When the above arrhythmias occur as a new event following a myocardial infarction the prognosis is very poor. This is due to the fact that they occur very often in response to pump failure, which in turn is usually due to a large infarct. With these arrhythmias, one often sees heart failure, hypotension and shock. These complications are due primarily to the underlying pathology and not the arrhythmia itself.

The modes of treatment mentioned above are designed to correct the arrhythmia only. The total treatment of pump failure of the heart involves many avenues of approach, which will be considered in a later chapter dealing with the complications of myocardial infarction.

E.   ARRHYTHMIAS OF ELECTRICAL FAILURE

The final type of arrhythmia is that due to electrical failure — ventricular fibrillation and asystole. This is the usual cause of sudden death when it occurs as a primary event following an acute MI. If there is time to do so, countershock is the obvious treatment for ventricular fibrillation, along with basic life support techniques. Asystole is treated by basic life support, advanced life support, and the insertion of a transvenous pacemaker. As a primary event following an acute MI, the salvage rate for both these arrhythmias is very low.

F. PACEMAKERS

No discussion of arrhythmias would be complete without some special consideration given to the use of pacemakers. The insertion of a transvenous pacemaker during the first 72 hours following an infarct (when the danger of arrhythmias is greatest) has become common practice in larger medical centers. This is done for specific indications only and has resulted in an improved survival rate in certain kinds of infarcts.

Indications for the use of a pacemaker are: An AV block of the Mobitz Type II or greater (including third degree heart block), a right bundle branch block with first degree heart block or left or right axis deviation, a bradycardia unresponsive to drugs, or a ventricular irritability with a slow rhythm. Justification for the use of pacemakers is that they will 1) decrease the incidence of Stokes-Adams attacks, 2) improve some cases of heart failure, 3) decrease the incidence of ventricular arrhythmias, and 4) enable the clinician to use strong antiarrhythmic medications and, in some cases, cardioversion.

Complications of pacemaker insertion are not common. The most common complication is a ventricular arrhythmia, and the physician inserting a pacemaker should have a defibrillator immediately available. Rare complications are perforation and sepsis.

Insertion of a transvenous pacemaker is rather simple. Sterile technique is required. After adequate preparation, the pre-packaged pacemaker electrode is inserted into any periferal vein that is accessible, although the physician may have a preference as to the site of insertion. The antecubital veins are usually chosen. The electrode is fed into the vein until it passes through the right atrium

and into the apex of the right ventricle. This
may be noted by using direct vision, using
the fluoroscope, or by attaching an ECG line
to the non-sterile end of the transvenous electrode and watching for the large typical ventricular complexes. The patient should be
connected to a cardiac monitor during the
entire procedure.

Before sterile technique is broken, the
pacemaker should be activated to check the
effective position of the electrode.

The use of pacemakers has increased
the survival rate in posterior inferior infarcts
by 22%.

The use and indications for indwelling
(surgically inserted) pacemakers is beyond
the scope of this book.

(The author was asked to add an Ap-
pendix to this Chapter, describing the diagnostic characteristics and standard treatment
of the common arrhythmias. This type of
cook-book approach to the coronary patient
is to be discouraged. We are not baking a
cake – we are treating a patient. This patient is different from all other patients we
will treat. We must follow certain rules and
guidelines if we are to prevent fatal arrhythmias, but we must do so with the knowledge
that this patient may react differently than
the others. We must diagnose promptly
(relying on a sound foundation and familiarity with cardiac physiology) and treat
the cause of the arrhythmia.)

CHAPTER 7

COMPLICATIONS
of
MYOCARDIAL INFARCTION

A. INTRODUCTION

The most common complication following a myocardial infarction is arrhythmia, and this has been discussed in the previous chapter. Power failure is the major cause of death in hospitalized post-infarction patients. Power failure connotes both heart failure and shock. Heart failure is a very serious complication, but can be treated successfully. Shock is a very ominous complication, and it has only been in the past few years that modern treatment has been able to influence its outcome. There are a number of surgical complications and some non-cardiac complications of myocardial infarction which will be discussed later in this chapter.

B. PUMP FAILURE

The term pump failure includes two distinct syndromes — heart failure and shock. It denotes a situation in which the heart is not performing its prime mission, as a pump, well enough to satisfy tissue perfusion demands.

There is a natural physiologic reserve that comes into play, when pump failure occurs. The normal arterial oxygen saturation is 97% and the venous oxygen saturation is 70% (this refers to mixed venous blood). When tissue perfusion is curtailed, as in pump failure, most vital tissues are able to extract a much higher percentage of oxygen. This is reflected by a lowering of the venous oxygen saturation. The lower limit at which oxygen demands can still be met is a venous oxygen saturation of 20%. It should be noted, that the heart and brain cannot make this type of adjustment. Both organs are extracting nearly maximal amounts of oxygen normally.

The cardiac index is a measure of the cardiac output as compared to the surface area of the body. The normal resting cardiac index is 3.0 liters/square meter. As was mentioned in an earlier chapter, there is always a decrease in the cardiac output following myocardial infarction. The cardiac index can go as low as $1.8L/m^2$ and still be sufficient to meet necessary perfusion requirements. In other words, the cardiac output can be decreased almost in half without damaging vital organs − if the cardiac output has not already been compromised by pre-existent disease.

Heart failure and shock will be considered as separate syndromes, but the treatment of the two has much in common, and the main points in the approach to their treatment are as follows:

1.   Correct arrhythmia to a sinus rate of 90 to 100.
2.   Correct hypovolemia to a normal CVP or wedge pressure.
3.   Correct hypoxia to an arterial oxygen saturation of 90% or greater.
4.   Correct pH and pCO_2 if abnormal.
5.   Improve cardiac contractility if necessary.
6.   Treat shock syndrome if necessary.

C.   HEART FAILURE

Left ventricular failure occurs in 63% of myocardial infarctions to one degree or another, and pulmonary edema in 16%. Congestive heart failure is a complex syndrome, and the precise explanation of each event in this syndrome is not completely understood. In heart failure following myocardial infarction, the basic pathology is in the left ventricle and the result is a decreased cardiac output. This results in a decreased renal blood flow and decreased glomerular filtration rate (GFR). By poorly understood mechanisms, the kidney then seeks to retain sodium (and along with the sodium, water). The result is fluid retention and an increased circulating blood volume. The greater blood volume increases the left ventricular filling pressure, which would thereby increase the cardiac output, by virtue of an increased stroke volume, in a normal heart. However, the infarcted ventricle is not normal and cannot increase its stroke volume. The result is a tachycardia and a continued increase in the diastolic filling pressure.

As the left ventricular end-diastolic pressure (LVEDP) increases there is a corresponding increase in the mean left atrial pressure and the pulmonary venous pressure. This is reflected clinically, by a rise in the pulmonary artery wedge pressure. Only after further advancement of the failure process, will the pulmonary artery, right ventricular and right atrial pressures rise. This is why a normal central venous pressure (CVP) is often misleading in accessing the function of the left ventricle.

The classical signs and symptoms of heart failure are generally related to an advanced state of this syndrome. Dyspnea is

106

shallow and rapid (as compared to the deep and slower respirations of the hyperventilation syndrome), <u>dyspnea</u> <u>on</u> <u>exertion</u>, <u>orthopnea</u>, left lateral decubitus dyspnea, and paroxysmal noctural dyspnea are all due to pulmonary vascular congestion and/or pulmonary edema. Cheyne-Stokes respiration and cough are also occasionally noted. As the failure progresses to involve the right side of the heart, there is systemic <u>edema</u>, starting first with dependent pedal edema and progressing to anasarca. As the abdominal contents become edematous there is ascites, painful swelling of the liver, anorexia, nausea, and abdominal distention. During the day there is <u>oliguria</u> and at night (or when recumbent) nocturia. Finally, there is inappropriate diaphoresis, fatigue and muscle wasting (due to the catabolic effects of chronically compromised perfusion).

The patient who has experienced recent rapid development of heart failure appears acutely ill, with dyspnea and perhaps diaphoresis. The chronic heart failure patient appears chronically ill with noticeable wasting. In either case, on physical examination, there may be cyanosis, diaphoresis, fine and coarse rales in the lungs as well as wheezing. The arterial pulse is rapid and responds to activity with an apparent inappropriate tachycardia. Pulsus alternans may be present. A Valsalva maneuver will have little effect on the peripheral pulse (as opposed to the normal response). The jugular venous pulse and the hepato-jugular reflex will be abnormal. On palpation, the heart is found to be enlarged, and on auscultation the <u>gallop</u> <u>rhythm</u> (third heart sound) is the hallmark of ventricular failure. A fourth heart sound may also be heard. A holosystolic murmur may mean poor apposition of the mitral or tricuspid valvular leaflets. An aortic systolic murmur may also be heard for the same reason.

The electrocardiogram is of little help in diagnosing heart failure, but the chest X-ray can be of great help.

Cardiomegaly (an enlarged heart) may or may not be present with heart failure, and when seen on the X-ray usually indicates a chronic process. The pulmonary radiographic changes in heart failure occur in degrees and, in the early stages, are rather subtle. The first change noted in heart failure is an enlargement of the pulmonary vessels. As the process progresses, there is a continued enlargement of the vessels in the upper lung fields, while the vessels in the lower lung fields become smaller. Normally, in the upright position, the vessels in the lower lung fields are larger due to gravity. The reversal of the normal situation is due to a reflex shunting of blood to the upper lungs. About this same time, one may note an increased prominence of the superior vena cava and azygos vein.

As failure continues to develop, interstitial edema occurs and the vessels become poorly outlined and foggy. This is referred to as hilar haze. At this stage in the process, one also notes Kerley Lines. There are three types of these. Kerley "B" lines are horizontal lines usually seen in the costophrenic angles. They are caused by thickening of the interlobular septa. Kerley "A" lines are vessel-like lines which go in the opposite direction from real vessels and are usually seen in the upper lung fields. Kerley "C" lines show up as a reticular pattern in the lower lung fields, but are rarely seen.

The next stage is caused by intra-alveolar edema, especially in the perihilar areas and is bilaterally symmetrical. This results in radiodensities in the inner and middle zones of the lungs which give a "butterfly" or "bat-wing" appearance to the hila on the X-ray.

108

The final stage of congestive failure in the lungs is pleural effusion. This seldom occurs with left ventricular failure alone, but almost always with biventricular failure. Pleural effusion can take one or more of several different forms. Effusion fluid in the free pleural space causes blunting of the costophrenic angle which can usually be seen on the PA projection. However, sometimes it is only visible on the lateral film. Effusion fluid may also accumulate in the interlobular fissures where they are seen as "pseudo-tumors". Finally, effusion fluid may collect in the subpleural space where it may simulate an elevated diaphragm. It should be noted that pleural effusions usually occur bilaterally, and sometimes only in the right lung, but seldom ever only in the left lung.

One should consider many factors before reaching a diagnosis of heart failure based on the chest X-ray. Pulmonary edema can be caused by non-cardiac conditions — such as drug addiction and on a neurogenic basis. If the heart size is normal, beware of the diagnosis of cardiogenic pulmonary edema. Any chronic lung disease will show an atypical pattern of congestive failure. Pleural effusion limited to the left lung is very likely not cardiac in origin.

The earliest and most reliable sign of heart failure is a rise in the wedge pressure.

In the treatment of heart failure, one can use the six point approach outlined earlier in this Chapter (page 105).

1.   All arrhythmias cannot be converted to a sinus rhythm. In the presence of heart failure, a bradyarrhythmia is first approached with IV atropine. If this is unsuccessful, an intravenous pacemaker should be inserted. With the restoration of an adequate

heart rate, there may be prompt reversal of the failure process.

Tachyarrhythmias can be considered a complication of heart failure and generally respond (if at all) to treatment of the underlying pathology. Specific treatment for these has been discussed in Chapter 6.

2. Correction of hypovolemia will be discussed at length later in this Chapter (in the section on Shock).

3. In the conscious patient, hypoxia can be treated with nasal oxygen or oxygen by mask. In the unconscious patient, other adjuncts must be used, including endotracheal intubation. See Chapter 11.

4. While the patient is receiving initial evaluation and treatment, blood gases and pH should be drawn and sent to the laboratory. After the results of these are known, appropriate therapy may be instituted. See Chapter 8. The efficacy of the oxygen therapy may also be evaluated.

5. Specific treatment for heart failure is discussed in the following pages.

6. In uncomplicated heart failure, there is usually no need to treat the shock syndrome.

There are two approaches to the treatment of congestive heart failure. One can attempt to reverse the renal contribution to heart failure by increasing the excretion of sodium and water through the kidneys by the use of diuretics. Or, one can approach the problem by treating the basic pathology, which is poor functioning of the left ventricle, with the use of a digitalis preparation to improve the contractility of the entire heart.

Most cardiologists recommend an approach to the basic pathology and the use of digitalis. There are a number of circumstances which modify this approach. In many instances the patient will already be fully digitalized, and the only approach to treatment of failure is by the use of diuretics. One should always consider the serum potassium when this is done. In acute pulmonary edema, one must use a rapid acting diuretic (ethacrynic acid or furosamide) and morphine sulfate intravenously, and digitalize later. If the patient is already taking both digitalis and a diruetic, rotating tourniquets and an increase in either or both of the medications may be in order. After the acute phase is over, both salt and water restriction must be considered.

Because of the acute nature of heart failure following a myocardial infarction, the speed of digitalization is of some importance. The most rapid acting, and least used, digitalis preparation is Ouabain. This drug can digitalize a patient within a matter of minutes but takes careful control by one experienced in its use. The most commonly used digitalis glycoside is digoxin (Lanoxin). It can be given IM, orally, or IV. The latter approach is recommended for rapid digitalization. Deslanoside (Cedilanid-D) is also quite useful for rapid digitalization. If necessary, diuretics may be added to the therapeutic regimen after digitalis has been started. This should only be done after careful monitoring of the serum potassium.

The digitalis glycosides and diuretics will be discussed fully in Chapter 9.

111

D.   SHOCK

Cardiogenic shock is the most serious non-surgical complication of myocardial infarction, with the exception of sudden death. It occurs in 15% of hospitalized infarct patients and carries a very ominous prognosis. It is due to a markedly decreased cardiac output — to the extent that the peripheral blood pressure and perfusion of vital organs cannot be maintained by the damaged left ventricle. Shock can also be viewed as a progressive metabolic disease that eventually reaches a point of irreversible damage to vital organs. It is characterized by a shift from aerobic to anaerobic metabolism with the production of lactic acid and acidosis. Early recognition and treatment is vital. The best treatment is prevention.

Shock, in general, may be due to three basic processes. The first is decreased venous return. This is seen in cardiac tamponade, constrictive pericarditis and hypovolemia. The second cause is decreased cardiac output as seen in myocardial infarction, valvular heart disease and cardiomyopathies. The third cause is from peripheral circulatory problems and is seen in toxic or septic shock. The first two types may be seen following a myocardial infarction.

The signs one sees with shock are due to the decreased arterial blood pressure and decreased tissue perfusion. Specifically, these signs are hypotension (systolic arterial pressure less than 90mm Hg or 30mm Hg below the previous basal level), urine output less than 20cc/hr, impaired mental functions, peripheral vasoconstriction (cold clammy skin and pallor). Shock due to pericarditis or cardiac tamponade is characterized by distended peripheral veins. In septic shock, peripheral vasoconstriction is usually

112

not seen. There is actually a peripheral vasodilation, and one notes warm dry skin. See Figure 7.1.

In cardiogenic shock, two subgroups are identified. The first group are those with shock on admission to the CCU. These are usually younger patients and the outcome is generally poor. The second group develop shock later in the course of their infarct and are usually represented by older patients. These patients usually take a steady downhill course and expire.

1.   Hypovolemic Shock

Hypovolemia literally means a decreased volume of fluid in the intravascular space. The most common non-cardiac cause of hypovolemia is hemorrhage. It can also be caused by fluid restriction with or without the concomitant use of diuretics, vomiting, diaphoresis, a shift of fluid to the extravascular compartment, or sepsis.

Simple hypovolemia and hypovolemic shock are different only in a matter of degree. They both present with hypotension. One should also be aware that hypotension does not always mean shock, and that hypotension in the cardiac patient may be due to other causes besides hypovolemia — such as a rhythm disorder, a vasovagal reaction, or as the effect of certain drugs (morphine sulfate).

When an acute cardiac patient presents in the emergency room or coronary care unit with hypotension, the first order of business is to determine the central venous or wedge pressure (preferably the latter). If the pressure is below the limits of normal or in the lower limits of normal,

113

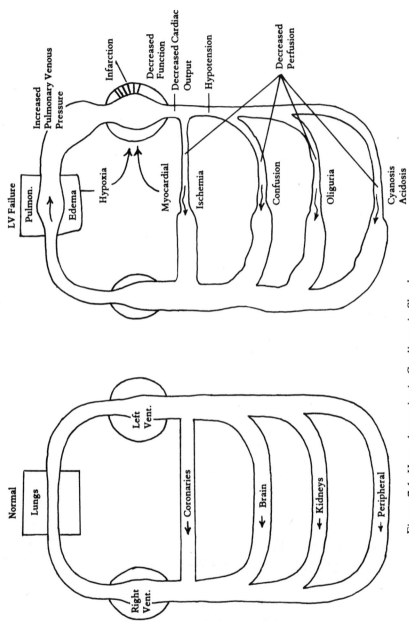

Figure 7.1 Hemodynamics in Cardiogenic Shock

114

a volume challenge is in order. A volume
challenge is the rapid infusion of intravenous
fluids (5% dextrose in water at the rate of
200cc in 10 minutes). If the problem is
hypovolemia, there may be a prompt increase in the blood pressure.

One may continue volume expansion
in this way until 1) there is an increase in
the blood pressure and decrease in the heart
rate or 2) there is an increase in the CVP
or wedge pressure to the upper limits of
normal. If 2) occurs and the blood pressure
is still low, one must look for another cause
for the hypotension besides hypovolemia.
It may be due to true cardiogenic shock
(pump failure), but it must be remembered
that patients with an acute MI may also be
septic or bleeding.

Some patients, who are volume chal-
lenged in this way, will show an immediate
rise in the CVP or wedge pressure and then
go into frank pulmonary edema. These are
the patients who were teetering on the brink
of pulmonary edema, and the challenge of
the additional circulating blood volume
pushed them over the edge. However,
this is not a disastrous situation. One
need only to withdraw an amount of fluid
from the CVP or PA line equal to that
which was infused to restore the previous
circulatory balance.

One should recall the warning mentioned in Chapter 2 concerning the basic
unreliability of the central venous pressure
in accessing left ventricular function. One
should also recall that even the wedge pressure is unreliable in patients with chronic
pulmonary vascular disease.

2.   Pump Failure Shock.

Shock due to pump failure and cardiogenic shock are basically synonymous terms. If the shock syndrome is still present after a trial of volume expansion, one must assume that, in the infarct patient, the cause is cardiogenic. Immediate treatment must be instituted.

Treatment of cardiogenic shock follows the same six points mentioned earlier.

1.   Correct arrhythmias as described in the section on heart failure.

2.   Correct hypovolemia, as described above, and maintain volume with 5% dextrose in .2% saline to keep the wedge pressure in the higher limits of normal (up to 18mm Hg). If the initial hematocrit is under 35%, whole blood may be used.

3.   Correct hypoxia as described in the section on heart failure.

4.   Shock is a state of anaerobic metabolism characterized by lactate production and acidosis. The acidosis should be treated by the respiratory route, if possible (using IPPB with a short positive pressure phase).

5.   If any signs of heart failure are present, rapid digitalization should be accomplished.

6.   Specific treatment for the shock syndrome is aimed at restoring and maintaining the arterial blood pressure. The systolic pressure should be maintained between 80—100mm Hg. Vasoactive drugs are essential for this type of treatment. The most commonly used drugs of this type are:

116

norepinephrine (Levophed, Levarterenol), methoxamine (Vasoxyl), metaraminol (Aramine), and dopamine. Dopamine seems to offer many advantages over the other drugs at the time of this writing. Isoproterenol (Isuprel) should never be used for cardiogenic shock due to its adverse effects on the myocardium. For a full description of these drugs and their mode of action, refer to Chapter 9.

An optional mode of treatment for the shock syndrome (from any cause, including cardiogenic shock) is with massive doses of corticosteroids (such as 1 gram of dexamethasone given IV). These high doses are used only for a few days, and seem to stabilize cellular membranes and prevent further cellular damage.

The counter-pulsating balloon pump is a recent innovation in the treatment of shock. It is the only mode of therapy which has significantly altered the discouraging course of this syndrome. The balloon pump is introduced surgically by catheter through one of the femoral arteries. It is fed up to the proximal aorta, and when connected to a control device which is synchronized with the electrocardiogram, inflates and deflates in unison with the natural left ventricular contractions. The result is a decreased afterload, an increased blood pressure, and improved perfusion of the coronary arteries.

E.   SURGICAL COMPLICATIONS

There are a number of surgical complications of myocardial infarction. The most serious is cardiac rupture, and is usually immediately fatal, due to cardiac tamponade or hemorrhage. It rarely occurs after three weeks following the infarct.

Septal perforation is a less serious complication and is heralded by the sudden onset of a loud apical systolic murmur. This usually occurs in the lower part of the ventricular septum, and is not associated with any ECG changes. The prognosis is good if the patient survives the acute infarction phase and gets to surgery. Right heart failure may be the predominant finding. Both of the above complications occur about ten days after the infarct, when the necrotic myocardium is the softest. The clinician must distinguish this condition from papillary muscle rupture.

During the convalescent period, one may also find the moderate systolic murmur of mitral insufficiency. This might be due to papillary muscle dysfunction which occurs in 15–20% of infarcts. It might also be due to rupture of a papillary muscle or chordae tendineae. The murmur must be distinguished from that of left ventricular failure and ventricular septal defect. Pulmonary edema is common with this condition. There is usually no precordial thrill. There is a very high mortality rate with rupture (80% in two weeks), but it is amenable to surgery if the patient survives the infarct.

Also during the convalescent period, several less acute complications may be encountered. Ventricular akinesis may occur. This happens when the scarred portion of the ventricle does not contract with the rest of the ventricle. If the scarred area is large enough, there will be a significant decrease in the stroke volume and perhaps heart failure. Ventricular dyskinesis is when the scarred part of the ventricle balloons out with each contraction. This, obviously, markedly reduces the stroke volume, since much of the work of the ventricle goes into the ballooned-out area. A ventricular aneurysm occurs when the ballooned-out portion

118

of the ventricle remains ballooned-out even during diastole. Ventricular dyskinesis or aneurysm should be suspected when there is a late onset of heart failure or shock. The heart failure is usually unresponsive to positive inotropes, such as digitalis. A persistently elevated ST segment is an important clue to these two conditions. A bifid pulse may also be noted. All three of the above conditions are amenable to surgical repair. If there is enough remaining myocardium to sustain an adequate stroke volume, and if the coronary artery disease is not too far advanced, the damaged area of the myocardium may be excised.

Acute pulmonary thromboembolism occurs rarely during the course of an infarction, if routine prophylaxis for this very serious complication is practiced. Precipitating factors incude 1) injury to the endocardium (as in a subendocardial or transmural infarct), 2) stasis, and 3) increased coagulability of the blood. X-ray findings of this condition are dilatation of the pulmonary artery and right ventricular enlargement but are rarely seen. ECG findings are those of right bundle branch block (RBBB) and decreased T waves in the anterior precordial leads (V1–V3), but these are usually absent. Clinical findings are the most significant information for the diagnosis. Central nervous system signs are very common and include anxiety, restlessness and syncope. Cardiac signs include heart failure, shock or arrhythmia. Pulmonary findings are pulmonary edema, wheezing and hypoxia. Cardiac output is reduced. Major findings are dyspnea and/or fever. Treatment consists of rapid anticoagulation (if this has not already been done), vena cava ligation, urokinase, and surgical removal of the clot.

Pulmonary infarction is seen rarely as a complication of heart failure, lung disease or shock. Other complications are pneumonia, post-myocardial infarction syndrome, and shoulder–hand syndrome. The reader is referred to a standard textbook for a description and diagnosis of these conditions.

F.   PROGNOSTIC SIGNS

In evaluating the infarct patient, certain signs may be used as prognostic indicators for eventual recovery.

Unfavorable signs are arrhythmias of pump failure (supraventricular arrhythmias, especially the tachyarrhythmias), complete heart block, and infarcts which affect both the anterior and posterior myocardium. Shock is a very unfavorable sign.

Favorable prognostic signs are a sinus bradycardia, absence of any arrhythmia (including ventricular irritability), and no signs of heart failure.

G.   LONG-TERM COMPLICATIONS

Pulmonary or systemic thromboembolism, in some series of post-infarction patients, occurs as often as 40–50% of the time. Pulmonary emboli make up 40% of the total.

Heart failure which occurs in the late convalescent period may be due to papillary muscle rupture or ventricular aneurysm or dyskinesis. Persistent angina may also be a problem. Arrhythmias may also occur during this period.

Of those patients released from the hospital following myocardial infarction, 40-50% will experience full recovery, 30–40% will have some reduction in activity, and 20% will be permanently disabled.

Follow-up care should include Stress Electrocardiograms at 3 months, 6 months, and one year (see Chapter 13). Intractable angina should be evaluated with coronary arteriography for the possibility of a saphenous vein bypass operation.

Before going home from the hospital, the patient should be counseled concerning 1) activity (including sexual activity) and occupation, 2) diet, 3) smoking, 4) alcohol, and 5) medications.

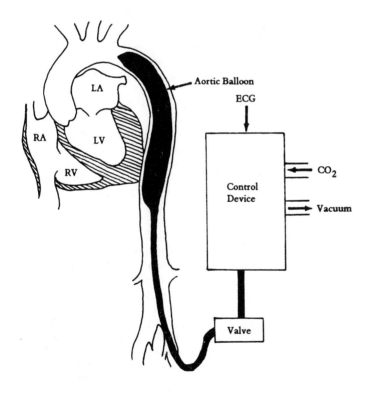

Figure 7.2   Counter-Pulsating Balloon Pump

CHAPTER 8

ACID-BASE BALANCE
and
ELECTROLYTES

A. INTRODUCTION

All metabolic functions of all living organisms are mediated and controlled by the workings of chemical systems, called enzyme systems. This is true of the human organism as well as other organisms. These enzyme systems control the normal functions of the kidneys, lungs, heart, liver, brain, and all the other organ systems of the body. Everything that happens in the body is caused by the proper functioning of one or more of these enzyme systems.

Like all chemical reactions, these enzyme systems work normally and properly only under certain conditions of heat and acidity. Each system has an optimal acidity at which it performs best, and this may be quite different for different parts of the body.

Normal metabolism is dependent on the ready supply of oxygen and yields carbon dioxide and water (as well as other chemicals) as the end products of this metabolism. This is called aerobic metabolism. If oxygen is not available, intracellular processes automatically shift to anaerobic metabolism which yields lactic acid as the end product. This occurs in shock or cardiac arrest. The lactic acid causes an increase in the acidity of the blood (drop in the pH) which is called acidosis, and this interferes with the normal function of many enzyme systems. When this occurs, compensatory mechanisms immediately come into play. The respiratory rate increases to expel more CO_2 from the lungs, and thus lower the acidity (and raise the pH). The kidneys retain HCO_3, which lowers the acidity, and raises the pH. However, the lungs and kidneys do this by the workings of their own enzyme systems which are also affected by the acidosis. Clinically, we step in to help restore the homeostatic balance by either hyperventilating the patient or giving intravenous bicarbonate, or both.

B.   MEASUREMENT OF BLOOD ACIDITY

Water (H_2O) consists of two ionizable particles – hydrogen ion (H^+) and hydroxyl ion (OH^-). Hydrogen ion carries a positive charge and will migrate to a negative electrode and is therefore called a cation (the negative electrode is called the cathode). The hydroxyl ion is negatively charged and migrates to the positive electrode (anode) and is called an anion. A solution of pure water contains as many hydrogen ions as hydroxyl ions and is called a neutral solution. When there is an excess of hydrogen ions over hydroxyl ions the solution is called acid or acidic. Where there is an excess of hydroxyl ions, the solution is called alkaline or basic.

Acidity, in the range of that which occurs in the body, is measured in pH. pH stands for the negative logarithm of the hydrogen ion concentration and can have a value of from 1 to 14. A pH of 1 would designate an extremely acid solution and a pH of 14 an extremely alkaline one. Water is directly in the middle, with a pH of 7. The normal pH of the blood is between 7.35 and 7.45 with an average of 7.4. Therefore, normal blood is slightly alkaline.

123

When the blood has a pH of less than 7.35 it is called acidemic and the condition called acidosis. Blood with a pH of more than 7.45 is alkalotic, and the condition called alkalosis.

The normal acidity of the blood is maintained by chemical systems called buffer systems. A number of these systems are in operation simultaneously. The largest of these systems is the hemoglobin-oxyhemoglobin system. The system which is of the most concern to us in normal clinical situations is the carbonic acid system. The reason for its importance is the ease by which it can be controlled by various clinical means and the ease by which its components can be measured in the laboratory. It also seems to be the natural system the body uses for rapid adjustments of the pH.

When carbon dioxide (CO_2) (which is a normal product of metabolism) is dissolved in water (which is the main component of the extracellular compartment and is also a product of metabolism) there is a chemical reaction as follows:

$$H_2O + CO_2 \rightleftharpoons H_2CO_3 \rightleftharpoons H^+ + HCO_3^-$$

This formula says simply that water (H_2O), when combined with carbon dioxide (CO_2) forms, and is in equilibrium with, a third compound, carbonic acid (H_2CO_3). The latter compound disassociates into two other substances — hydrogen ion (H^+) and bicarbonate ion (HCO_3^-). In other words, all five of these substances are co-existent, and three of them can be readily measured in the laboratory (CO_2, H^+ and HCO_3^-).

There is a mathematical relationship between hydrogen ion, carbon dioxide and bicarbonate ion, so that in fact we only need to know two in order to calculate the third. This relationship is expressed by the following formula:

$$[H^+] = \frac{K \times p CO_2}{[HCO_3^-]}$$

$[H^+]$	Hydrogen ion Conc.
K	A constant
pCO_2	Partial pressure CO_2
$[HCO_3^-]$	Bicarbonate Conc.

In situations which cause minor deviations in bicarbonate or carbon dioxide (such as eating very acid food) the carbonic acid buffer system absorbs the excess of one by increasing the other, and maintains the pH in the normal range.

When there is a deviation in the pH of the blood it must obviously be either to the acidotic side (pH less than 7.35) or to the alkalotic side (pH greater than 7.45). Two organ systems usually maintain the carbonic acid buffer system in a homeostatic balance. The respiratory system maintains the proper amount of carbon dioxide in the blood by excreting excess carbon dioxide through the lungs. The kidneys dispose of excess bicarbonate by excreting it through the urinary tract. When both organ systems are functioning properly, minor deviations in the pH are corrected rapidly.

Major deviations in the pH are conveniently classified as either respiratory or metabolic — meaning that the acidosis or alkalosis is due either to dysfunction of the respiratory tract or dysfunction in metabolism of the entire organism or the kidneys alone.

125

Respiratory acidosis is due to chronic (and sometimes acute) lung disease or holding the breath, and expelling less CO_2 than normal. Carbon dioxide and hydrogen ion are increased and the pH lowered. Respiratory alkalosis is due to hyperventilation — breathing off too much CO_2 — and is treated by sedatives or re-breathing expired air (to raise the CO_2). The carbon dioxide and hydrogen ion are lowered and the pH increased.

Metabolic acidosis can be due to a variety of disease states, such as diabetes, cardiac arrest, shock, toxic ingestions, etc. Treatment is directed at the underlying disease along with Ringer's solution, bicarbonate, etc. The bicarbonate and pH are lowered and the hydrogen ion elevated. Metabolic alkalosis can be due to gastric suction or too forceful treatment with diuretics. This is frequently associated with a low serum potassium and chloride. Treatment is with rapid replacement of chloride ion in the form of chloride solutions. Potassium replacement must be done more slowly with the use of potassium chloride (KCl) at the rate of 10mEq/hour. Potassium replacement without concomitant replacement of chloride is seldom indicated. One can also use acetazolamide (Diamox) which blocks the enzyme system in the kidneys causing the re-absorbtion of bicarbonate. Bicarbonate and pH are both increased and the hydrogen ion decreased.

To review briefly, the first line of defense for variations in the blood pH is the buffer systems. These systems are of brief and limited value. The second line of defense is the compensatory mechanisms — the lungs and the kidneys. When the compensatory mechanisms take effect, the formulas and changes in the laboratory values are not so clear-cut, and we then derive new syndromes – "compensated" respiratory acidosis, or "compensated" metabolic acidosis, etc. This situation is further complicated by the fact that one may find "mixed" acidosis or "mixed" alkalosis, meaning that there is a metabolic and respiratory component to the problem. Figure 8.1 is a nomogram of blood acid-base balance. By inserting the laboratory values into the nomogram, one may determine the cause of the acid-base disturbance. Many laboratories will report blood gas analysis, pH, and bicarbonate on such a form, thus saving the clinician time in figuring out the problem. One should also not forget that the clinical picture can be the most valuable information in determining an acid-base imbalance.

The results of the blood gas and pH determinations may be reported in terms of base excess (BE) or base deficit (BD). This relates to the amount of bicarbonate ion necessary to restore the normal equilibrium. A primary metabolic acidosis always results in a base deficit. The amount of bicarbonate necessary to restore equilibrium is gotten from the formula: weight (in Kg) times the BD times .3. The result of computation gives the mEq of bicarbonate needed. If the acidosis is acute, the entire dose is given at once. If it is chronic (compensated), one-half is given. A primary metabolic alkalosis always results in a base excess.

When the pCO_2 and base deficit or excess move in the same direction (from normal) a compensating effect has taken place. When they move in opposite directions, a mixed acid-base problem is present.

In the past, before the ready availability of blood gases and pH from the modern laboratory, the clinician attempted to extrapolate the above information from other lab-

127

oratory tests — HCO_3^-, Cl^-, CO_2 content, CO_2 combining power, serum sodium and potassium. The conclusions drawn from these tests were sometimes accurate but often misleading. With the current ready access to pH, pCO_2, pO_2, and HCO_3^- from the laboratory, one can make an accurate determination of the pH problem and its cause.

Normal values for acid-base and electrolyte parameters are given in Table 3.

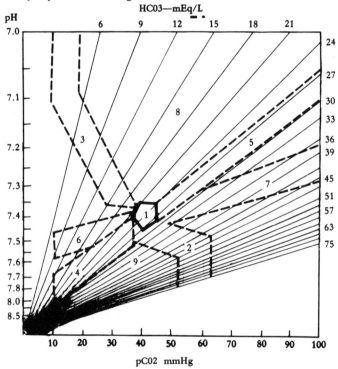

1. Normal
2. Metabolic Alkalosis
3. Metabolic Acidosis
4. Respiratory Alkalosis
5. Respiratory Acidosis

6. Compensated Resp Alk
7. Compensated Resp Acid
8. Mixed Acidosis
9. Mixed Alkalosis

Figure 8.1   Acid-Base Nomogram

C. ELECTROLYTES

The body can arbitrarily be divided into three compartments: the intracellular compartment which is the tissue contained within the cells, the interstitial compartment which is the tissue between the cells, and the intravascular compartment which is the fluid in the circulatory system (this includes all arteries, veins, capillaries, and the blood in the heart chambers. The interstitial compartment and the intravascular compartment can be combined into another compartment called the extracellular compartment. The logic for doing this is quite simple. The constituents of these two compartments are very similar, but quite different from the intracellular compartment.

Acid-base disturbances are often associated with electrolyte disorders. Electrolytes are particles which when dissolved in solution carry an electric charge. Sodium chloride (NaCl, salt) when dissolved in water is an electrolyte. In water, the two parts of the compound, sodium and chloride, dissociate into sodium ion (Na^+) and chloride ion (Cl^-). The sodium ion carries a positive charge and the chloride ion a negative charge. They are both electrolytes. Electrolytes are usually measured in the blood in terms of milliequivalents per liter (mEq/L). Equivalency refers to chemical activity.

Other chemicals, when dissolved in water, do not dissociate and gain an electric charge. These chemicals are called non-electrolytes and are usually measured in the blood in terms of milligram percent (milligrams in 100ml of serum) or mg% or mg/100ml. Examples of non-electrolytes are glucose, creatinine, urea, and alcohol.

129

The total number of dissolved particles in a solution, whether they be electrolytes or non-electrolytes is measured in terms of osmolality (the force of osmotic pressure through a semipermeable membrane) and expressed as milliosmoles per liter (mOsm/L). Osmolality is essentially synonymous with tonicity. An isotonic solution is one with the same osmolality as body fluids. Hypertonic solutions have a higher osmolality and hypotonic solutions a lower osmolality than body fluids. In larger laboratories the osmolality is measured directly by an osmometer. In smaller laboratories, it is estimated by the serum sodium determination. The normal plasma osmolality is 300mOs/Kg. This is roughly twice the numerical value of serum sodium, and can be estimated as such.

The principal electrolytes in the blood are sodium ion (Na^+), chloride ion (Cl^-) and bicarbonate ion (HCO_3^-). The principal intracellular electrolytes are potassium ion (K^+), sulfate ion (SO_4^-) and phospate ion (PO_4^-).

NORMAL VALUES

pH	7.35-7.45		
pCO_2	38-42 mmHg		
HCO_3^-	24-27 mEq/L		
BE	$\pm$ 2		
pO_2 (room air)	80 mmHg		
	70 (in older patients)		
pO_2 (100% O_2)	600 mmHg		
Cl^-	96-106 mEq/L		
K^+	3.5-5.0 mEq/L		
Magnesium	1.5-2.5 mEq/L	Calcium	9-11 mg%
Na^+	136-145 mEq/L		4.5-5.5 mEq/L
Phosphates	3-4.5 mg%		
Sulfates	.8-1.2 mg%		

Table 3. Normal Blood Gas & Electrolyte Values

D.   RENAL COMPENSATORY MECHANISMS

Before we consider how the kidneys
react to alterations in the pH and electrolyte
balance, we must first examine the way the
kidneys function normally. The functioning
unit of the kidney is the nephron. There are
approximately one million of these nephrons
in each normal kidney. The first part of the
nephron is the glomerulus. It is a fine network of arteriolar capillaries. The vessel leading into the glomerulus is the afferent arteriole
and the vessel leading from it is called the ef-
ferent arteriole. Each glomerulus is surrounded by a sac, called Bowman's capsule. This
leads to the tubular part of the nephron.

As the blood passes through the glomerulus, the hydrostatic pressure of the blood is
greater than the osmotic pressure of the plasma proteins and the interstitial pressure of
the capillaries. Therefore, a certain part of
the fluid portion of the blood is filtered
through the capillary wall into Bowman's
capsule. The filtered fluid is called the
glomerular filtrate. In the normal adult, the
amount of this filtrate is approximately 100
ml/minute. The rate of formation of the
filtrate is called the glomerular filtration
rate (GFR).

Approximately 99% of the filtrate will
be returned to the circulation by tubular reabsorption. The other 1% will be excreted.
After the filtrate leaves Bowman's capsule,
it drains into the proximal convoluted tubule,
the descending limb of Henle's Loop, Henle's
Loop, the ascending limb of Henle's Loop,
the distal convoluted tubule, a collecting
duct, and then to the more distal portions
of the drainage system, and finally excretion.

Refer to Figure 8.2

131

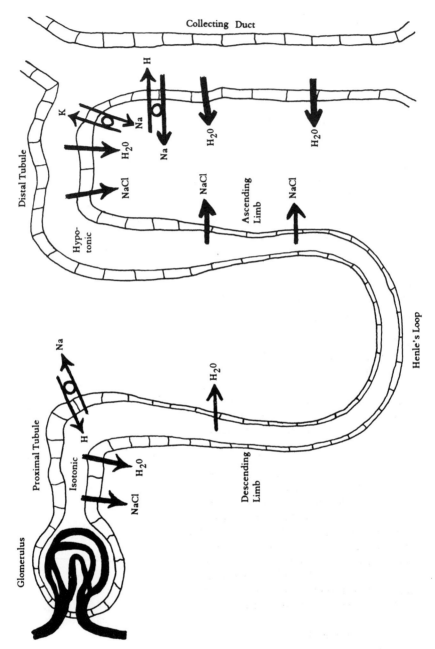

Figure 8.2   The Nephron

132

During its trip through the nephron, many things happen to the filtrate changing it from an ultrafiltrate of plasma into urine. In the proximal tubule, approximately 60 to 70% of the filtrate is reabsorbed and much of it as isotonic sodium, chloride and water. Also in the proximal tubule, all the potassium and about 90% of the bicarbonate is reabsorbed. An additional amount of sodium ion is reabsorbed here in exchange for hydrogen ions from the tubular cells. This reaction is made possible by the enzyme carbonic anhydrase which catalyses the reaction of carbonic acid to give hydrogen ion and bicarbonate ion.

In the descending limb of Henle's Loop, additional water is reabsorbed. In the ascending limb, 15 to 30% of the filtered sodium is reabsorbed, but since this part of the nephron is relatively impervious to water, an equal amount of water is not reabsorbed, and the urine at this point becomes hypotonic. In the distal tubule, the remaining 8 to 10% of the filtered sodium and bicarbonate is reabsorbed. Much of the sodium in the distal tubule is reabsorbed in exchange for potassium and hydrogen ions which are actively secreted into the tubular fluid. This reaction is called the sodium pump. Also in the distal tubule, hydrogen ions combine with ammonia to form ammonium ion (NH_4^+), and with HPO_4^- to form H_2PO_4 (the latter is called titratable acid).

In the collecting duct, there is additional reabsorption of potassium (which was secreted along with hydrogen ion in the distal tubule), and water.

The total amount of acid eliminated in the urine is equal to titratable acid plus ammonium ion less the amount of bicarbonate not reabsorbed. Normally, ammonium ion accounts for two-thirds of the excreted acid and titratable acid for only one-third.

From the above, it can be seen that the kidney maintains acid-base balance by two mechanisms; the carbonic anhydrase reaction and ammonium ion production. The carbonic anhydrase reaction turns CO_2 and water into bicarbonate and hydrogen ion. The bicarbonate ion is reabsorbed as sodium bicarbonate and the hydrogen ion goes on to combine with HPO_4^- to form titratable acid. Ammonium ion production relies on the enzyme glutaminase which catalyses the reaction of glutamine (an amino acid biproduct of protein metabolism) to glutamic acid and ammonia (NH_3). Ammonia freely diffuses across the tubular cell membrane and in the tubular lumen combines with hydrogen ion to form NH_4^+.

Respiratory acidosis is characterized by a lowered pH and high CO_2 (called hypercapnia or hypercarbia). In chronic respiratory acidosis, the kidneys react by secreting more hydrogen ion (as ammonium ion and titratable acid), and this results in generation of more bicarbonate. The combined result is to maintain the pH at 7.4. In acute respiratory acidosis, there is little renal compensation. The treatment is by forced hyperventilation.

Respiratory alkalosis is a result of hyperventilation and causes a low CO_2 (hypocapnia or hypocarbia) and a low pH. Here the renal threshold for bicarbonate excretion is lowered so that bicarbonate appears in the urine. Normally, 100% of bicarbonate is reabsorbed. The treatment is sedation or by use of a rebreathing bag.

The renal responses to changes in pCO_2 take place entirely in the proximal tubule. The direct secretion of hydrogen ion takes place in both the proximal and distal tubules. The proximal tubule has a great capacity for secreting hydrogen ion but can do so only against a small gradient. On the other hand, the distal tubule has a much smaller secretion capacity but can do so against a much larger gradient.

After an initial response of the respiratory center to increase the ventilatory rate (and thus decrease CO_2), the kidneys respond to metabolic acidosis by secreting more hydrogen ion and thereby increase the HCO_3^- which was initially reduced by the buffering system action. Acute metabolic acidosis is characterized by a sharp decrease in both bicarbonate and CO_2. As the condition becomes more chronic, there is a smaller reduction in both. The treatment of metabolic acidosis has been discussed in other chapters.

Metabolic alkalosis results from too vigorous gastric suction or protracted vomiting or from diuretics. In this condition, there is a concomitant loss of sodium, potassium and chloride ions. The renal response to this condition tends to sustain the alkalosis. The patient has lost large quantities of hydrogen and chloride ions, causing a decrease in the serum H^+ and Cl^- and an increase in HCO_3^-. He has also lost large quantities of Na^+ and K^+ ions. The kidneys attempt to restore homeostasis to the extracellular fluid by retaining sodium at the expense of excreting K^+ and H^+, and this worsens the alkalosis and the hypokalemia. The immediate treatment is with chloride ion as sodium chloride (NaCl) since the sodium will effect a bicarbonate diuresis. It is equally important to replace the potassium ion to correct the acidosis since the distal tubule will continue to secrete hydrogen ion in the presence of hypokalemia. This must be done more slowly

135

(usually as KCl at the rate of 10mEq/hour).
Acetazolamide (Diamox) can also be used to
block the reabsorption of bicarbonate.

In the next chapter we will consider
the effects of diuretics on these renal mechanisms. Let us now consider the effects of
other physiologic and pathophysiologic
processes.

There is a small organ next to the glomerulus called the juxtaglomerular apparatus.
This organ is sensitive to any change in the
arteriolar pressure. If the pressure drops, the
juxtaglomerular apparatus secretes the hormone Renin, which in turn causes the formation of Angiotensin I and then Angiotensin II
from precursors in the plasma. Angiotensin II
causes the secretion of Aldosterone from the
adrenal cortex, and this hormone causes increased reabsoprtion of Na+ in exchange for
K+ and H+ in the distal tubule. Abnormally
high levels of this hormone (hyperaldostero-
nism) results in hypokalemia, hypernatremia,
and alkalosis.

Antidiuretic hormone (ADH) is secreted
by the posterior lobe of the pituitary gland in
response to increased osmolality of the blood.
ADH is also secreted in response to hypotension. This is mediated through the barorecep-
tors in the carotid sinus and the ninth cranial
nerve. Pain, emotional stress, morphine, volume depletion and decreased cardiac output
also enhance the secretion of ADH. Increased
ADH causes increased water reabsorption in
the tubules.

Renal blood flow is approximately 25%
of the total cardiac output at rest. This
amounts to a renal blood flow of roughly 1.5
liters per minute. This results in a GFR of
100-120 ml/min. (and a total volume of
urine of 500-2000 ml/day. Hemodynamic
factors are an important influence on renal
function, and this is especially true in the
cardiac patient. Decreased renal blood flow
results in decreased GFR and oliguria. Urine
production may be used as a rough estimate

of renal blood flow. The critical level of urine production which represents adequate blood flow to meet nutritional needs of the kidneys is 20 ml/hr.

The GFR can be determined by the Creatinine Clearance in the laboratory. The normal GFR decreases with aging so that by age 60 the normal GFR is 50-60 ml/min. The Creatinine Clearance depends on the muscle mass of the body and is fairly constant. From Figure 8.3, it can be seen that there must be a significant decrease in the GFR before there is a noticeable decrease in the Creatinine Clearance.

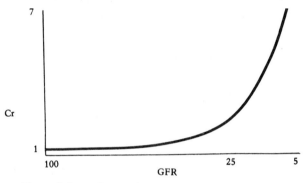

Figure 8.3   Serum Creatinine

An acute decrease in renal blood flow results in the secretion of Renin, Angiotensin I & II, and Aldosterone. The latter causes the retention of sodium. If there is also a decrease in blood pressure (as in shock), ADH is produced causing a retention of water.

A similar effect is seen in heart failure. Sodium is retained and along with it, water. In this case, the retention of both sodium and water is inappropriate and worsens the heart failure. Because of the added effect of ADH, and possibly other mechanisms, water is retained in excess of sodium so that hyponatremia develops. At a serum sodium of 116 mEq/L, generalized seizures may be seen. The treatment for this degree of hyponatremia is immediate infusion of 200cc of 3% NaCl.

137

The clinician should not forget that there are other causes of oliguria besides pre-renal causes (hypovolemia, hypotension, decreased cardiac output). These are called post-renal and consist of prostatic hypertrophy and other obstructive uropathy. All the above causes of oliguria are reversible, but there is a large group of irreversible causes which have to do with permanent kidney damage and must be treated with dialysis. The rule of thumb in renal failure is to dialyse early before toxicity develops.

Cardiac patients are prone to several fluid and electrolyte disturbances either from their heart disease or their therapy. We have already considered the mechanisms of salt and water retention in heart failure. The initial treatment for this is restriction of dietary salt and the judicious use of diuretics. Water need be restricted only in those patients who develop a hyponatremia. Hyponatremia in the heart patient is always due to too much water, not to too little salt.

A low serum potassium (hypokalemia) is a serious condition which can cause life threatening arrhythmias. Its effects are additive to those of digitalis, so that a normal dose of digitalis in the presence of hypokalemia can cause digitalis toxicity. Hypokalemia in the cardiac patient is usually due to the use (or overuse) of diuretics. It is usually associated with a low serum chloride and sometimes alkalosis. Hypokalemia can be diagnosed from the electrocardiographic criteria of depressed and shortened ST segment and a prominent U wave. A prolonged QT interval may or may not be present. See Figure 8.4. The treatment is discussed above.

Hypokalemia is associated with both ventricular and supraventricular tachyarrhythmias and with PVCs.

138

Hyperkalemia (high serum potassium) may occur in the cardiac patient due to decreased delivery of sodium to the distal tubule and subsequent decreased exchange of potassium for sodium. There also may be increased reabsorption of potassium in the collecting ducts. Hyperkalemia will result in cardiac toxicity by causing depolarization of the membranes and thus interferes with normal depolarization. Electrocardiographic changes include low P waves, prolonged PR interval, prolonged QRS (AV nodal and intraventricular blocks) and a tall, peaked and narrow T wave. See Figure 8.5.

Mild hyperkalemia can be treated by restriction of potassium intake, avoidance of potassium-sparing diuretics and increase of dietary sodium (to increase potassium excretion). Severe hyperkalemia is a true medical emergency and is treated by intravenous sodium bicarbonate to cause a shift of potassium into the intracellular compartment. Cardiac toxicity may be avoided by intravenous calcium gluconate (10-30cc of 10% solution over 1-5 minutes). One must be very careful however in doing this on a digitalized patient. After the acute phase is over, a longer term shift of intracellular potassium may be had with intravenous hypertonic glucose and insulin (10 units). Later, potassium exchange resins, either orally or as an enema, may be used. Dialysis may be necessary in some cases of severe hyperkalemia.

When we measure the serum potassium, what we are really interested in determining is the total body potassium — both intracellular and extracellular. The principal intracellular cation is potassium ion. If the serum potassium is normal or high, we can make no estimates as to the total body potassium, since a high potassium may rep-

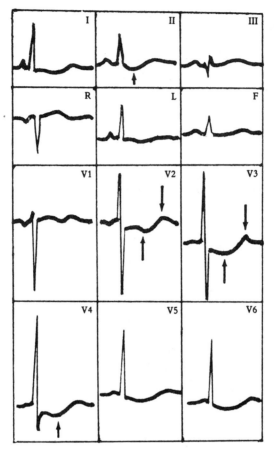

Figure 8.4 Hypokalemia

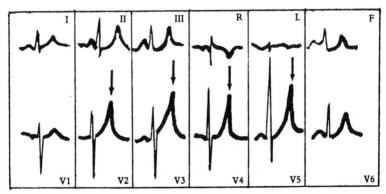

Figure 8.5 Hyperkalemia

140

resent a shift of potassium out of the cells and into the blood. In the same way, a normal serum potassium may not reflect a cellular deficit of potassium. However, when the serum potassium is low, we may conclude that the total body potassium is also low.

An abnormal serum calcium can have a profound effect on cardiac function. Calcium metabolism is regulated by parathyroid hormone and Vitamin D. The rate of gastrointestinal absorption and renal excretion is fairly constant in the normal individual. The largest portion of calcium is excreted in the gastrointestinal tract. Tubular reabsorption of calcium is nearly 100%. In renal tubular disease, unusual amounts of calcium may be lost, resulting in hypocalcemia. This produces muscular hyperirritability, tetany and convulsions. Cardiac effects include diminished contractility with prolongation of the ST segment and QT interval. The T wave is lowered. If cardiac arrest occurs due to hypocalcemia, it occurs in diastole. See Figure 8.6.

Hypercalcemia may result from over secretion of parathyroid hormone, hypervitaminosis D, or too vigorous treatment with calcium. Systemic symptoms include muscular flaccidity, weakness and stupor. Cardiac effects include increased contractility, PVCs and idioventricular rhythms. Electrocardiographic changes include a shortened QT interval, absent ST segment and an abruptly ascending T wave close to the R wave. With severe hypercalcemia, cardiac arrest occurs in systole. See Figure 8.7.

Although serum calcium disturbances are not often seen in the acute cardiac patient, their prompt treatment when they are present is crucial. The immediate treatment

141

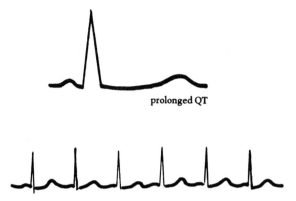

prolonged QT

Figure 8.6 Hypocalcemia

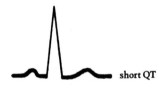

short QT

Figure 8.7 Hypercalcemia

of hypocalcemia is intravenous calcium gluconate given in one gram increments slowly. Extra care and cardiac monitoring are necessary if the patient is also receiving digitalis. Hypercalcemia is treated in the acute situation with hydration and potassium and sodium replacement (they are both usually low) and with glucocorticoids.

Hypochloremia is often associated with hypokalemia and alkalosis (see above). The treatment is rapid replacement of chloride ion.

Hypomagnesemia (low serum magnesium) can occur in many situations including diuretic therapy. A chronic magnesium deficiency results in reduced intracellular potassium. Digitalis likewise causes a reduced intracellular potassium. It stands to reason that if a patient has been on diuretic therapy (and suffered a loss of both magnesium and potassium) digitalis toxicity may develop readily. The treatment is by infusion of magnesium sulfate (2-6 cc of 25% solution).

Lactic acidosis is the result of shock. The treatment for this has been considered elsewhere. It should be stressed that acidosis depresses cardiac output in a range of 7.2 to 7.25 pH. At a pH of 7.1 the heart is no longer able to react normally to catecholamines.

In addition to the renal effects described above, Angiotensin is also a potent arteriolar vasoconstrictor and thus raises the blood pressure.

E.   PULMONARY COMPENSATORY MECHANISMS

The function of respiration is to supply the body with an adequate oxygen gradient and to remove carbon dioxide. This involves

143

three very different processes. The first is ventilation — the delivery of oxygen-rich atmospheric air to the innermost part of the lung — the alveoli. The second process is diffusion which is the movement of oxygen through the alveolar wall and capillary wall into the blood, and the reverse course for carbon dioxide. The third process is circulation of the oxygen-rich and carbon dioxide-poor blood to the cells of the body where the opposite exchange takes place (oxygen leaves the blood and carbon dioxide enters). Diseases of any of these three processes interferes with proper respiration. In the cardiac patient, all or any of the three can be affected.

Ventilation is accomplished so effortlessly in the normal individual that one hardly is aware of it happening. The respiratory muscles (intercostal and diaphragm) contract, expanding the chest and lowering the alveolar pressure to less than the atmospheric pressure. This causes air to flow into the lung. In expiration, the muscles relax and the chest contracts, thus raising the intra-alveolar pressure, and forces the air from the lungs. Expiration is an entirely passive process, except in patients with chronic obstructive lung disease. These patients have to force the air from the lungs in expiration.

Diffusion of gases in the lung is compromised by any increase in the alveolar or capillary walls or the interstitial tissue between the two. This is seen in interstitial fibrosis, pulmonary edema or lung infections. Acute pulmonary edema is often associated with a mixed acidosis. As compensation occurs, a respiratory acidosis is found. In diffusion problems, one does not usually see an elevated pCO_2, but a low pO_2 is noted. This is because CO_2 diffuses across the alveolar-capillary bridge readily while O_2 has much more difficulty doing so. The primary central nervous stimulant to increased respiration is an elevated CO_2. Hypoxia is a secondary stimulus to respiration and the pO_2 must get very low before respiration is significantly influenced. As the perfusion abnormality becomes severe, the CO_2 will eventually rise above normal.

Circulation problems are those of the general circulation (such as congestive heart failure which causes a respiratory alkalosis) and those peculiar to the lung. The latter are referred to as ventilation-perfusion abnormalities. These occur either by altered alveolar ventilation or by abnormal alveolar capillary perfusion. For instance, if an alveolus is poorly ventilated but receives a normal capillary perfusion, the blood leaving that alveolus will not be normally oxygenated. Or, if a normal alveolus receives less than normal capillary perfusion, the blood leaving it again will be low in oxygen. Pulmonary function tends to deteriorate in the first three days following acute infarction in otherwise uncomplicated cases. Ventilation-perfusion difficulties are the cause of this. The most severe cases of decreased pulmonary function are those patients with pulmonary edema or segmental atelectasis.

Alveolar hypoventilation refers to the condition in which the alveoli do not receive enough atmospheric air to afford proper exchange of oxygen and carbon dioxide. This syndrome may be seen with diseases of several organ systems − brain, spinal cord, chest wall, upper and lower airways, and the heart. The symptoms and signs of this syndrome are those of hypercapnia and hypoxia. The symptoms of the former are listed in Table 4, and the latter in Table 3. The signs of both are rather non-specific. The arterial

pCO_2 is an indicator of alveolar ventilation
and any increase in it means alveolar hypoventilation. Hypoxemia may be due to
many causes. It is also possible for the patient to have a high pCO_2 and a normal
or even elevated pO_2 if he is receiving oxygen
(as is the custom with myocardial infarction).
In this case, the patient would show the signs
of CO_2 narcosis without the signs of hypoxia.

Respiratory failure may occur sudden-
ly or incidiously following myocardial infarction. The shallow respirations following pain,
fright, or morphine sulfate may accentuate
the pathologic problems in the lungs, and lead
to alveolar hypoventilation. The clinician
must be alert to the signs of respiratory failure
and institute appropriate therapy. Acute respiratory failure is most common in patients
with chronic pulmonary disease, but is also
seen with pulmonary emboli and congestive
heart failure.

The primary treatment of acid-base
disturbances, hypercapnia or hypoxemia due
to pulmonary function is with controlled or
assisted ventilation, with or without oxygen.
Ventilation therapy can also be a second line
of defense in metabolic acid-base problems.
The manner in which this is done depends
on the condition of the patient. The unconscious patient must have an airway inserted
and receive at least ventilatory assistance (if
he has spontaneous respirations). The conscious patient may need positive pressure devices, hyperventilation, or a rebreathing device. In any case, after ventilatory therapy
has been started, the blood gases and pH
must be monitored constantly to maintain
the proper gas and pH balance.

Before leaving the subject of pulmonary compensatory mechanisms, it should be mentioned that the amount of CO_2 which is blown off during ventilation (and measured by the pCO_2) is not the only CO_2 which is gotten rid of during the normal ventilatory cycle. A certain amount of new CO_2 is formed from bicarbonate ion by the enzyme carbonic anhydrase (the same enzyme we found earlier in the kidney). This enzyme is also involved in the elaboration of cerebrospinal fluid and the aqueous humor of the eye.

Poor Judgment	Restlessness
Fatigue	Impaired Motor Function
Confusion	Dizziness
Delirium	Tachycardia
Central Cyanosis	Warm extremities
Hypotension	Unconsciousness

Table 3.   Signs of Hypoxemia

Headaches	Sweating
Dizziness	Confusion
Asterixis	Miosis
Papilledema	Tachycardia
Hypertension	Gastric distention
Shock	Arrhythmia

Table 4   Signs of Hypercapnia

CHAPTER 9

CARDIAC DRUGS

A. NON-CARDIAC DRUGS

This section will deal with drugs that are used in heart disease and myocardial infarction, but do not have any direct cardiac effect.

1. Anticoagulants

In years past, anticoagulants were employed in acute myocardial infarction with the idea that they would prevent extension of the infarct. This is now known not to be true. However, anticoagulants are quite useful in preventing one of the major complications of forced absolute bed rest – thromboembolism. Thromboembolic disease is fairly common in low output states (such as myocardial infarction) and can account for more prolonged morbidity than the primary disease. The emboli usually originate in the lower extremities or pelvis. This complication can be prevented, in most cases, by the use of anticoagulants along with other preventive measures.

Anticoagulation is not without hazards and must be used judiciously. It should not be used in the presence of any bleeding or if there is a potential of bleeding. Some cardiologists use it only with younger patients or with first infarctions. Others use it with older patients or with severe infarcts. Many use it with women patients and with congestive heart failure.

Heparin is the first line of treatment for anticoagulation because of its immediate onset of action. It neutralizes thrombi and inhibits Coagulation Factors IX and XI.

148

When using Heparin, the Lee-White Clotting Time must be monitored at least daily *, and in some cases more often, to insure an effect between the therapeutic range and the dangerous range. The therapeutic range is to prolong the Clotting Time to two or three times the normal. A Clotting Time between 30 and 35 minutes is usually adequate for effective anticoagulation. The dosage schedule is noted below. The IV route is preferred in acute myocardial infarction. The effects of Heparin are blocked by antihistamines.

Method	Frequency	Dose
Subcutaneous	Every 8 hours	10,000 units
	" 12 "	15,000 to
		20,000 units
Intramuscular	" 8 "	10,000 "
Intermittent IV	" 4-6 "	10,000 "
		fol by 5-10,000
Continuous IV		20-40,000 units/
		day in 1000cc sol.

Warfarin (Coumadin, Panwarfin) and bishydroxycoumarin (Dicumarol) are anticoagulants used in the convalescent period following an infarction. These substances compete with Vitamin K and thereby interfere with the synthesis of Factors VII, IX, and X. They also inhibit the synthesis of prothrombin, and their therapeutic effect is controlled clinically by following the Prothrombin Time. The therapeutic range is 20-30% of the control. These drugs are not necessarily used in every infarct patient during convalescence and are of little benefit after six to eight weeks.

Drug	1st Day	2nd Day	Maintenance
Dicumarol	200-400mg	100-200mg	100mg
Coumadin	30-50 mg	10-15 mg	7mg

* The Activated Clotting Time (ACT) can be used.

149

2. Nitrites

Nitroglycerine has been the standard of treatment for angina for decades. Isosorbide dinitrate (Isordil, Sorbitrate) is a newer drug with essentially the same effects. Their action is on smooth muscles and especially the muscle layer of venules. This results in venodilatation, decreased venous return, decreased blood pressure, increased heart rate, decreased stroke volume and ejection time, and decreased heart size. The sum total effect is a decreased myocardial oxygen consumption. There is also a decreased cardiac output, which is of no consequence if the original cardiac output was adequate to insure effective perfusion pressure in the coronary arteries. However, if the original perfusion pressure was only marginal, a further lowering may worsen the cardiac state. It was originally thought that the nitrites reduced angina by causing widespread vasodilatation in the coronary bed. This is now known to be untrue, but the nitrites will relax spasm in the coronary vessels.

If nitroglycerine is combined with an alpha-adrenergic stimulator, the adverse blood pressure and heart rate effects of the nitroglycerine are reversed, and a definite salutary effect is seen, even two hours after total occlusion of the coronary artery. Propranolol may also be combined with nitroglycerine, and their effects are complementary. Nitroglycerine also seems to enhance electrical stability during ischemia.

The current status of nitroglycerine in the treatment of acute myocardial infarction is undecided. It is not a part of the routine therapy.

3. Oxygen

Of all drugs that have been used in the treatment of myocardial infarction, oxygen is the most common.

150

Oxygen is carried in the blood by two separate mechanisms. Part of it is combined with hemoglobin to form the compound oxy-hemoglobin. This is the compound that makes arterial blood redder than venous blood. The amount of oxy-hemoglobin in the blood is measured by the oxygen saturation. The normal individual, when breathing room air, will have an arterial oxygen saturation of 90 to 98%. With the breathing of 100% oxygen, this is raised to 99 to 100%. This, obviously, is not a significant increase in oxygen saturation.

However, a large amount of oxygen is dissolved in the blood. When breathing room air the amount of oxygen dissolved in the blood is .3cc per 100 cc of plasma (or expressed as partial pressure, 100mm Hg). The breathing of 100% oxygen will raise this amount of dissolved oxygen to 1.8 cc per 100 cc plasma (600mm Hg). This sixfold increase is quite significant and is the rationale for the use of oxygen in myocardial infarction. It is assumed that by increasing the oxygen content of the blood the injured and ischemic myocardium adjacent to the infarct will be able to survive.

The normal partial pressure of oxygen (pO_2) is greater than 80mm Hg in arterial blood or 70mm Hg in older patients. The critical level which represents a significant decrease in the pO_2 (and usually the cardiac output) is 60mm Hg. The most efficient means of delivering oxygen is at 100% with the intermittent positive pressure breathing machine (IPPB). Oxygen has also been found to lower serum lactate.

Like all drugs, oxygen therapy is not without significant complications. When delivered at high pressure (in the range of 3 to 4 atmospheres) convulsions can occur.

151

The use of positive pressure oxygen can result in a "wash-out" of nitrogen from the lungs, minor obstructive phenomena, focal atelectasis, and a right to left shunt of blood which lowers the pO_2. Frequently, large inhalations are helpful in preventing this series of events (sighing at the rate of 5 per hour).

As the pO_2 increases with therapy, there is a direct depressant effect of the myocardium and an increase in the heart rate. A continued pO_2 of 500mm Hg can lead to over-hydration, pulmonary edema and peripheral edema.

It should be noted that in all instances of myocardial infarction, there is a decrease in arterial pO_2. This is felt to be due to focal areas of atelectasis. This decrease is, of course, much more pronounced with pulmonary edema or segmental atelectasis (collapse of a portion of the lung).

Several studies have shown no change in the mortality rate following myocardial infarction with the use of oxygen.

4.   Narcotics

Pain and apprehension is a common finding in most cardiac patients. Traditionally, morphine sulfate has been used to allay both pain and anxiety. It is a most valuable drug. Besides relieving pain, it also produces a state of euphoria. Unfortunately, it also causes a decreased blood pressure and respiratory depression, when given in the usual therapeutic doses of 10 to 15 mg. These adverse side effects are not noted with smaller doses (3 to 4.5 mg) given intravenously every 5 to 30 minutes. It has also been shown that morphine sulfate increases the blood flow to the heart and brain.

152

Meperidine (Demerol) is a good anal-
gesic, but it does not have the euphoric effect of morphine. It does not reduce the
blood pressure as much as morphine. Tal-
win has been used with myocardial infarctions, and when given in adequate doses,
seems to relieve pain as well as Demerol,
without causing a decreased blood pressure.
In some instances, the blood pressure is increased.

5.   Sedatives

Sedatives have commonly been used
to treat infarction patients. They allay a
certain amount of anxiety and assist in
keeping a normally active patient at bed
rest.

The barbiturates have little or no
cardiovascular or respiratory effects in the
usual doses given for daytime sedation.
However, these compounds depend on a
normal renal blood flow for the predicted
excretion rate. If the renal blood flow is
decreased (as in heart failure or shock),
a rapid toxic level of these drugs may
build up and have a strong depressant effect on the central respiratory center.

Barbiturates have been abandoned in
favor of the tranquilizers. The commonly
used tranquilizers do not cause cardiovascular or respiratory depression. Meprobamate and Valium are effective skeletal
muscle relaxants, as well as tranquilizers,
but do not appreciably affect the blood
pressure. They are both used widely following myocardial infarction.

Night-time hypnotics may be used
in the infarct patient if there is no danger
of toxic build-up. The most commonly
used drug in this category is chloral hydrate,

which is metabolized mainly in the liver and some of the by-products excreted through the kidneys.

6. Bicarbonate

Sodium bicarbonate is used during emergency cardiac care (ECC) to counteract the acidosis of anaerobic metabolism during anoxia. In the past, it was given every 10 minutes until cardiac function was restored or until the patient expired. However, it has been found that multiple doses of bicarbonate are not without significant side effects. With increasing doses, the blood osmolality rises to levels which can be fatal. In hospitals that have an osmometer, the osmolality can be measured directly. If this machine is not available, one can make a close estimate of the osmolality by measuring the serum sodium. This should not be allowed to go over 155-160 meq/L. Metabolic alkalosis can also occur from too vigorous bicarbonate therapy. The serum sodium, blood gases and pH should be determined on admission and again after the second dose of bicarbonate. The results of these tests should be considered before the third dose of bicarbonate is given. If any of these results are in the dangerous range, further treatment for the acidosis should be by forced ventilation to a pCO_2 of 25-30mm Hg.

7. Fluids

Intravenous fluids are required to some extent during every myocardial infarction, especially during the acute phase when rapid delivery of anti-arrhythmic drugs or Heparin may be necessary. At other times, the IV lines, CVP line or PA line must be kept open. The most commonly used fluids are 5% dextrose in water or 5% dextrose in .2% saline.

154

Fluids are essential in the correction of hypotension due to fluid depletion (as discussed in Chapter 7). Great care must be exercised in monitoring the total fluid balance to prevent volume overload. This is done by watching the central venous or wedge pressure. Another parameter to consider is the urinary output. The fluid input can be titrated to a urinary output of no less than 20cc/hr.

8. Diuretics

Before considering the action of the diuretics, the reader is requested to review the section in Chapter 8 on renal compensatory mechanisms. Each of the five classes of diuretics interferes in some way with the reabsorption of sodium (and its attendant anion and water). Each class of diuretic has its own type of effect and its own way of disturbing electrolyte and acid-base balance. These imbalances should not, however, be considered toxic effects of these drugs, since these imbalances represent the expected way in which these drugs work.

Mercurial diuretics are the oldest and still the most effective natriuretic agents. Their exact site of action is still unknown, but they effectively inhibit tubular reabsorption of sodium and chloride. Even though they inhibit the Na-K exchange in the distal tubule, a large mercurial diuresis can result in hypokalemia. The distal tubular exchange of Na-K is not inhibited, and may even be enhanced. The result of these many separate actions can lead, in some patients, to a hypokalemic alkalosis. This can be prevented (and the efficacy of the diuretic enhanced) by the concomitant use of ammonium chloride. See Figure 9.1. These diuretics cannot be given orally.

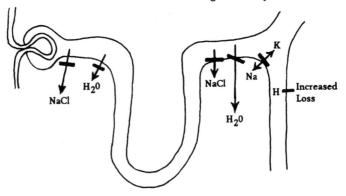

Figure 9.1   Action of Mercurial Diuretics

Carbonic anhydrase inhibitors were the first effective oral diuretics. They inhibit the formation of hydrogen ion from carbon dioxide and water in the proximal and distal tubules and thereby reduce sodium and hydrogen exchange through the nephron. These drugs produce a significant sodium bicarbonate diuresis and a loss of potassium. A hyperchloremic metabolic acidosis may develop. The effects of the carbonic anhydrase inhibitors antagonize the effects of the mercurial diuretics, but enhance the effects of the thiazides, ethacrynic acid and furosemide. The most commonly used drug in this class is acetazolamide (Diamox).
See Figure 9.2.

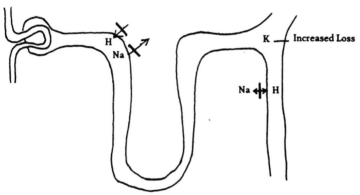

Figure 9.2   Action of Carbonic Anhydrase
              Inhibitors.

The thiazide diuretics are chemically related to the sulfonamides and are the most commonly used oral diuretics. They may be given both orally and parenterally. They depress the glomerular filtration rate and thereby induce azotemia in some patients. They are potent inhibitors of tubular reabsorption of sodium and also interfere with dilution of the urine, and can lead to dilutional hyponatremia. Sodium-potassium ion exchange in the distal tubule is accelerated by these drugs and a hypokelemia and metabolic alkalosis

157

can be produced by their continued use. Low oral doses also produce a hyperuricemia and can provoke acute gouty arthritis. See Figure 9.3. There is a plethargy of this type of drug on the market, and the reader is referred to the PDR for standard dosages and administration.

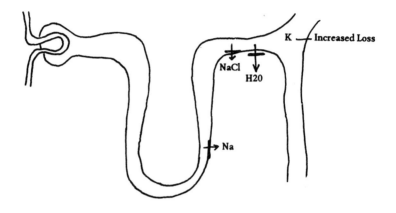

Figure 9.3   Action of Thiazide Diuretics.

Potassium-sparing diuretics were introduced to combat the hypokalemic side effects of the thiazide diuretics, and at this time, the most commonly used forms of these drugs are combined with a thiazide. There are basically two kinds of these preparations and both antagonize the effects of Aldosterone. Spironolactone (Aldactone; with a thiazide it is called Aldactazide) only antagonizes the Aldosterone effects. Triamterene (Dyrenium; called Dyazide when combined with a thiazide) not only antagonizes the action of Aldosterone, but produces a sodium diuresis and reduces potassium and hydrogen ion loss even in the absence of Aldosterone. These drugs are much more effective when combined with other diuretics. Side effects include azotemia, hyperkalemia (in patients with kidney disease), and hyponatremia (in edematous patients). See Figure 9.4.

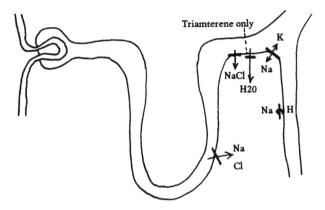

Figure 9.4   Actions of Spironolactone
              & Triamterene.

Ethacrynic acid and furosemide are the newest and most potent diuretic agents. They are thought to act in the Loop of Henle, and for this reason are referred to as the "loop diuretics". They produce a significant sodium diuresis, along with moderate amounts of potassium and chloride. They may often produce diuresis in a patient who is unresponsive to other diuretics, but their effect is somewhat unpredictable and should be used with much caution. These compounds can also lead to hypokalemia and metabolic alkalosis. They work well when combined with one of the Aldosterone antagonists. See Figure 9.5.

Intermittent therapy of one to three days, and combinations of several types of diuretics seem to produce a greater diuresis in the refractory patient.

Most of the above mentioned diuretics can cause a hypokalemia and this may provoke digitalis toxicity in patients receiving the latter drug. One can use potassium supplements prophylactically to prevent this complication, but hyperkalemia is then possible. The safest method for the use of diuretics in the acute situation is by the constant monitoring of the serum electrolytes and subsequent replacement on a calculated basis. One should also be aware that when potassium is lost through the urinary tract, it is almost always combined with chloride ion, and if replacement is necessary, <u>both</u> ions must be replaced. There are a number of potassium supplements on the market that do not contain chloride ion. These are not recommended.

The most common use of diuretics in the myocardial infarction patient is with acute pulmonary edema or exacerbation of heart failure. There is another use of furosemide which should be mentioned. In a low output state (such as shock), there may be a very low urinary output for prolonged periods of time. In order to "flush the kidneys", an intravenous dose of Lasix may be given. The fluid lost by this method is immediately replaced intravenously to maintain the circulating blood volume.

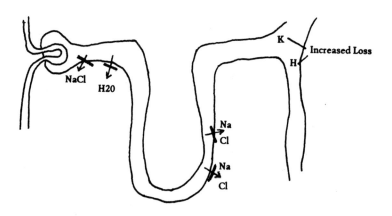

Figure 9.5   Action of Loop Diuretics.

B.   ANTIARRHYTHMIA DRUGS

An understanding of the action of antiarrhythmic drugs presupposes an understanding of the electrophysiology of the cardiac
cellular membrane during the cardiac cycle.
We are most concerned with three properties
of cardiac tissue – automaticity, conduction
velocity and the refractory period. These
three properties are due to the movement of
sodium and potassium across the cellular membrane. During diastole, the negative intracellular charge is maintained by the action of the
enzyme adenosine triphosphatase (ATPase)
which keeps potassium in the cell and sodium
outside the cell. In pacemaker cells, this action is incomplete and some sodium manages
to get into the cells thus reducing the transmembrane potential. This is called diastolic
depolarization and accounts for pacemaker
activity.

With depolarization, sodium rushes into the cell rapidly changing the negative intracellular potential to a positive charge. This
occurs during the QRS phase of the ECG, and
the speed with which it occurs is related to
the conduction velocity. During repolarization (the refractory period), potassium leaves
the cell to restore the negative potential in
the cell. This occurs during the QT interval.
During the resting phase (diastole), potassium
is pumped back into the cell and sodium is
pumped out by the action of ATPase.

Calcium transport across the cell membrane is also a factor in the cardiac cycle.
The contractile force of the myocardial fibers
is influenced by this transmembrane movement
of calcium. Positive inotropic agents enhance
the movement of calcium across the membrane while negative inotropes reduce it.

It is currently felt that arrhythmias
are the result of either one or the other of

161

two processes. The first is increased automaticity and is due to excessive diastolic depolarization in an ectopic cell. This leads to a repetitive discharge and propagation and an arrhythmia such as ventricular tachycardia.

The second process causing arrhythmia is a result of altered conduction velocity and refractory period. This results in reentry phenomena and circus movements (See Chapter 6). This is felt to be the most common cause of arrhythmia in coronary artery disease.

All drugs used for arrhythmia control reduce diastolic depolarization and thus automaticity. All of these agents effect the refractory period and most of them act upon the conduction velocity. Those antiarrhythmic drugs that lengthen the refractory period and reduce the conduction velocity are classified as Type I drugs. Those that shorten the refractory period and speed conduction velocity are Type II. Figure 9.6.

Quinidine and procainamide (Pronestyl) are the most commonly used Type I antiarrhythmics. They bind to the cell membrane and prevent the ready movements of cations across it. By decreasing the ease by which sodium passes across the membrane during depolarization, they decrease the conduction velocity. By reducing the ease by which potassium leaves the cell during repolarization, they lengthen the refractory period. Finally, they decrease sodium entrance into the cell during the resting phase and this decreases diastolic depolarization and automaticity. By the above effects, these two drugs increase the PR interval and the duration of the QRS complex. These drugs also have an anticholinergic action (like atropine) which

162

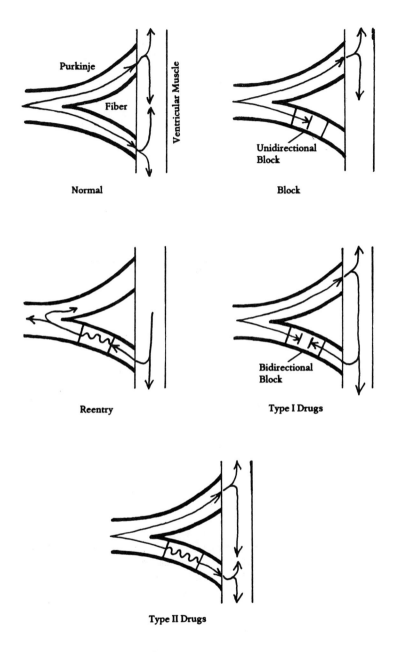

Figure 9.6 Mechanism of Action of Antiarrhythmics

163

may augment or oppose the direct action
noted above. They are both negative inotropes and also decrease the peripheral resistance and blood pressure. These drugs
should not be used in the presence of any
heart block (without a pacemaker in place),
and the patient should be digitalized before
their use. Both are excreted in the urine,
so great care must be exercised when the
urine output is compromised.

Quinidine is given in doses of 200 to
400 mg every 6 hours orally or intramuscu-
larly. It is given intravenously at the rate of
25 mg/minute to a total of 800 mg. Procainamide is given every 6 hours at a dose of 250
to 500 mg, orally or IM. Intravenously, it is
given as 100 mg every 5 minutes to a total of
1 gram. Clinical indications for the use of
these two drugs are atrial fibrillation, atrial
flutter, paroxysmal supraventricular tachycardia, and PVCs. The gastrointestinal side
effects of quinidine often preclude its use.
These include nausea, vomiting, and diarrhea.
Procainamide can then be used with good
results, but should not be continued for
long periods in high dosage due to the lupus-
like syndrome it may cause.

Propranolol (Inderal) is a beta-adrener-
gic blocking agent and has a strong negative
inotropic effect. Because of this latter property, it has been used successfully in angina
which has been refractory to usual modes of
treatment. By reducing the strength of myocardial contractions, the work load and oxygen demands of the heart are reduced. In dog
studies, Inderal has been shown to reduce the
size of the infarct, even though it causes a
coronary vasoconstriction. Inderal lowers the
blood sugar and is contra-indicated in heart
failure and asthma.

In the treatment of arrhythmias, Inderal

164

has two significant effects: a direct quinidine-like effect which decreases automaticity and conduction velocity (however, the refractory period is shortened), and an indirect or beta-blocking action. This latter effect reduces sympathetic stimulation to the myocardium and thereby decreases conduction velocity, and automaticity and increases the refractory period. The influence on the refractory period goes along with the dominant effect.

Propranolol is most useful in treating supraventricular tachyarrhythmias which are not digitalis induced. It is also useful in the treatment of digitalis induced ventricular tachyarrhythmias. The oral dosage of Inderal is 10-30 mg every 6 to 8 hours. It may be given IV with an initial dose of 1 to 3 mg not to exceed .1 mg/Kg/24 hours.

Bretylium is an infrequently used Type I antiarrhythmic because its effects are some-times rather unpredictable. It causes the re-lease of norepinephrine from nerve endings and then blocks norepinephrine transmission. It can initially cause an increase in PVCs, after which it exerts a potent antiarrhythmic effect. It is given in doses of 350 to 400 mg IV, and can also be given orally.

Lidocaine (Xylocaine) is a Type II anti-arrhythmic drug even though it is similar in chemical structure to quinidine and procain-amide. It has no effect on sodium transport during depolarization and thus has no effect on conduction velocity, and will not induce or worsen heart block. It enhances potassium escape from the cell, and thus shortens the refractory period. Like all antiarrhythmics, it does decrease automaticity by reducing the rate of sodium entrance into the cell dur-ing the resting phase.

Lidocaine has no significant cardiovas-cular side effects, but does have some rather disturbing central nervous system effects, such as convulsions and coma, when given in high doses or for prolonged periods of time. It is usually given in a bolus of 50 to 100 mg intravenously, followed by an IV drip of 1 to 4 mg/minute. The real advantage of this drug is its immediate onset of action as an antiarrhythmic.

Diphenylhydantoin (Dilantin) is the other Type II antiarrhythmic. It enhances the movements of sodium and potassium across the cell membrane during depolarization and repolarization and thus speeds conduction velocity and shortens the refractory period. Like the other antiarrhythmics, it decreases automaticity by slowing sodium transport during the resting phase. This drug is useful in both atrial and ventricular tachyarrhythmias, but is most useful in those which are digitalis induced because it will not induce or worsen heart block. It is metabolized in the liver, so that renal clearance is not a problem. It is generally used when the standard antiarrhythmics have proved ineffective. It is given intravenously in the dose of 100 mg every 5 minutes until the desired effect is noted or until a total dose of 1 gram is given. It is given orally in the dose of 100 mg every 6 hours.

It has been demonstrated that arrhythmias due to reentry phenomenon and circus movement may be abolished by either shortening or lengthening the refractory period and increasing or decreasing the conduction velocity. Clinically, we do not know whether a given arrhythmia is due to this mechanism or due to ectopic automaticity. A reasonable approach is to try one or two of the Type I drugs and if unsuccessful go on to the Type II drugs. However, one should not ignore the specific indications for the Type II drugs (PVCs or VT with Lidocaine or digitalis

toxicity with Dilantin). One should also remember that potassium chloride is a power-
ful antiarrhythmic in the presence of hypokalemia. Countershock is a last resort treatment
for many tachyarrhythmias when the above
medications prove ineffective. There has been
much concern regarding the use of countershock when the patient has been digitalized
because of the possible emergence of ventricular tachyarrhythmias. This danger may be
minimized by using only a small voltage for
initial countershock and increasing the voltage in a stepwise fashion, as needed. Atrial
pacing is another alternative for the treatment
of digitalis induced arrhythmias.

Although atropine is not truly an antiarrhythmic drug, it is used in the treatment
of bradyarrhythmias associated with hypotension because of its parasympathetic blocking effects. See Chapter 6 for a full description of its actions. It may be given in doses
of .5 to 1 mg orally, intravenously or intra-
muscularly every 4 to 6 hours. Side effects
are a dry mouth and blurred vision. Toxic
effects include fever and psychosis. It is
contraindicated with glaucoma. It may cause
urinary retention and therefore must be used
with caution in older male patients (unless
a catheter has been inserted).

Digitalis glycosides have numerous effects on the heart. They are the drugs of
choice for heart failure but are also quite useful for certain types of arrhythmias. In this
section, we will consider only their use for
the latter. Digitalis compounds are effective
in supraventricular arrhythmias by the workings of two mechanisms – by direct action
on the conduction system and by reflex action through the vagus nerve.

There are basically three direct actions
of digitalis. The first is to slow AV conduction. This leads to increasing degrees of heart

167

block when block is present. This effect is seen on the ECG as a prolonged PR interval. The second effect is prolongation of the refractory period in the AV node. This effect results in slowing of the ventricular rate in supraventricular tachycardias. A third effect is seen only with toxic doses of digitalis, and consists of enhanced automaticity of the entire conduction system, except the SA node. This can lead to serious ventricular arrhythmias.

By reflex vagal stimulation, digitalis reduces the rate of pacemaker activity in the SA node.

Digitalis effects on the transmembrane action potential depend on the dosage used. In usual therapeutic doses, the duration of the action potential is increased due to a prolongation of Phase 3. This explains the first two direct effects noted above. In higher doses, there is a shortening of the action potential with a specific decrease in Phase 2 and/or Phase 4. The latter results in an increased rate of diastolic depolarization and explains the enhanced automaticity with toxic doses of digitalis.

In addition to the prolonged PR interval, other ECG changes may be noted with digitalis. A characteristic depression or sagging of the ST segment is often seen. This depression has a "scooped-out" appearance. The QT interval may be shortened and there may be inversion of the T wave.

Toxic effects include many gastrointestinal symptoms and many types of arrhythmias: Sinus bradycardia, AV dissociation, atrial and ventricular tachycardia and AV block, etc. These arrhythmias may be due to digitalis or to the underlying heart disease. This is only one of the reasons that digitalis should only be used when absolutely necessary.

A direct pressor effect (increased blood pressure) can sometimes be noted after the injection of one of the rapidly acting digitalis compounds.

As an antiarrhythmic, digitalis is indicated in all arrhythmias of pump failure (atrial flutter and fibrillation; sinus, atrial, and nodal tachycardias) and in intractable ventricular arrhythmias accompanied by heart failure.

The salutary effects of the Foxglove plant for the treatment of "dropsy" has been known since the late 18th century when William Withering described it. It was somewhat later that digitalis leaf was prepared from the plant extract. There are a number of plants and at least one animal (a toad) from which the digitalis glycosides may be extracted. The many digitalis preparations differ in their dosage, speed of onset, excretion and duration of action. Their therapeutic effects are all the same. See Table 5.

Although a standard adult dose has been established for all the digitalis preparations, the digitalizing dose for any given patient may be quite different from this. The clinician must individualize the dosage in each case. Certain cautions in the use of digitalis are well established: the full digitalizing and maintenance doses are reduced in older patients, in patients with congestive heart failure and in patients with impaired renal function. A full digitalizing dose does not have to be given before therapeutic effects are noted. The dose of digitalis when used as an antiarrhythmic may be many times the standard dose.

DRUG	DIGITALIZING ORAL	DOSE IV	MAINTENANCE DOSE
Digitalis Leaf	1.2-1.5 gm		100 mg
Digoxin (Lanoxin)	2-3 mg	1-2 mg	.25 –.5 mg PO
Lanatoside C (Cedilanid)	6 mg		1 mg
Deslanoside C (Cedilanid –D)		1.2-1.8 mg (6-8 ml)	
Ouabain		.5 mg	

Table 5.   Digitalis Preparations

DRUG	DOSAGE	INDICATIONS	COMPLICATIONS
TYPE I DRUGS			
Quinidine	200-400 mg IM, PO 25 mg/min IV to a total of 800 mg	Premature Contractions Atrial arrhythmias	Most toxic of group. May induce arrhythmias. Danger of hypotension.
Procainamide (Pronestyl)	250-500 mg IM, PO 100 mg q 5 min IV to total of 1 gm	Same as Quinidine Must give on 3 hr schedule.	
Propranolol (Inderal)	1-3 mg initial IV to total of 10-15 mg.	Supraventricular arrhythmias Good in combination with other drugs	Negative inotrope (heart failure) Bronchospasm
Bretylium	3-5 mg/Kg IM, IV q8-12 hours. 300-600 mg q8-12 hr PO	Refractory Ventricular arrhythmias	
Potassium	40mEq IV in no less than 2 hours (KCl)		

Table 6.   Antiarrhythmics

171

DRUG	DOSAGE	INDICATIONS	COMPLICATIONS
TYPE II DRUGS			
Lidocaine (Xylocaine)	50-100 mg IV fol by 1-4 mg/min	Ventricular irritability	CNS Stimulation
Diphenyl-hydantoin (Dilantin)	100 mg q 5 min to total of 1 gm IV	Digitalis toxicity Quinidine, procainamide toxicity	CNS Depression

Table 6 (cont'd)

C.   DRUGS USED IN HEART FAILURE

The therapeutic use of digitalis in the treatment of arrhythmias has already been discussed. The major role of digitalis is in the treatment of heart failure. All digitalis preparations have a strong inotropic effect and directly affect the myocardium to strengthen myocardial contractions. Digitalis has little effect on the normal myocardium, and indeed, has little effect on the failing heart that is not enlarged. It exerts its principal beneficial effect on the enlarged failing heart. In this latter situation, increased strength of myocardial contraction results in increased stroke volume and increased cardiac output.

This salutary effect is not without a price. With increased strength of contractions goes an increased oxygen consumption. This can have deleterious effects on the damaged or ischemic myocardium and can actually extend the infarct. The increased oxygen demands caused by digitalis are not nearly as pronounced as with isoproterenol.

Digitalis is thought to exert its positive inotropic effect by enhancing the movement of calcium across the cell membrane during depolarization.

Diuretics are sometimes used as the initial treatment of low-grade heart failure. They are often combined with digitalis in the treatment of more advanced failure. The actions of the diuretics have been discussed earlier in this chapter. These drugs are mentioned now only to warn against the danger of electrolyte imbalance when both drugs are used concomitantly. The use of potassium supplements is helpful in this respect.

173

D.   DRUGS USED IN CARDIOGENIC SHOCK

Until the 1950s, shock was treated almost exclusively by replacement of fluids and other supportive measures. In the early 50s, the unique properties of the catecholamines were applied to the treatment of shock and have been used, in varying degrees, for this condition ever since. Various terms have been used for these compounds – pressor amines, pressor substances, sympathomimetic amines, etc. The action of the sympathetic nervous system has been considered in Chapter 2. These drugs cause activation of sympathetic reserves in the heart and vascular system.

Sympathetic nervous system effects may be divided into two types: alpha adrenergic and beta adrenergic. Alpha stimulation results in what has traditionally been called the "pressor effect". See Figure 9.7. The smooth muscles used in the "fight or flight" reaction are contracted. Contraction of the venous and arterial smooth muscles causes an increase in the peripheral resistance and increased blood pressure. Increased venous pressure enhances diastolic filling and thus an increased cardiac output and blood pressure. However, the vasoconstriction also causes decreased tissue perfusion. Cardiac effects include positive inotropism and coronary vasodilatation. When the peripheral resistance is quite high, there may be a decreased cardiac output and heart rate even with the positive inotropism. An alpha blocking agent (such as Dibenzyline) will interfere with the smooth muscle contractions, but will not block the cardiac effects.

Beta stimulation of the adrenergic receptor sites causes a relaxation of smooth muscle, and specifically the smooth muscle of the arterioles. This results in decreased peripheral resistance and decreased venous pooling, which, in turn, results in increased cardiac output. The blood pressure may be

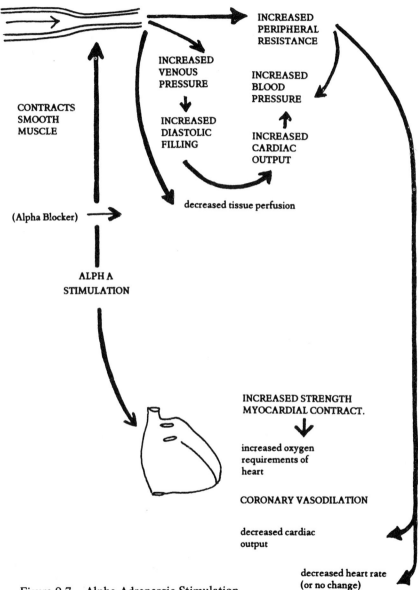

VENOUS & ARTERIOLAR
VASOCONSTRICTION

INCREASED
PERIPHERAL
RESISTANCE

INCREASED
VENOUS
PRESSURE

INCREASED
BLOOD
PRESSURE

CONTRACTS
SMOOTH
MUSCLE

INCREASED
DIASTOLIC
FILLING

INCREASED
CARDIAC
OUTPUT

decreased tissue perfusion

(Alpha Blocker)

ALPHA
STIMULATION

INCREASED STRENGTH
MYOCARDIAL CONTRACT.

increased oxygen
requirements of
heart

CORONARY VASODILATION

decreased cardiac
output

decreased heart rate
(or no change)

Figure 9.7   Alpha Adrenergic Stimulation.

lowered to dangerous perfusion levels. Depending on many factors, increased venous pooling may result which will lower the cardiac output.

Beta effects on the heart are both positive inotropic and positive chronotropic (increased strength of contractions and increased heart rate). Both of these result in increased cardiac output. But both effects also increase the oxygen demands of the myocardium, and in the presence of a myocardial infarction, can extend the area of necrosis. This is the reason that the purest beta stimulator, isoproterenol, is contraindicated in acute infarction. Arrhythmia is an added complication of beta stimulation. The beta effects on the heart may be blocked by propranolol (Inderal). See Figure 9.8.

The catecholamines occur as natural substances at sympathetic nerve endings throughout the body and are liberated by stimulation of the nerve. In addition, epinephrine and norepinephrine are released into the general circulation by the adrenal gland in conditions of severe stress. The sequence of synthesis, storage and release of the catecholamines is as follows: Phenylalanine ⟶ Tyrosine ⟶ DOPA ⟶ Dolamine ⟶ norepinephrine ⟶ epinephrine.

The last four substances, in the above list, have therapeutic usefulness in clinical medicine. DOPA (in the form of alphamethyldopa) is used in the treatment of hypertension. Dopamine, norepinephrine, and epinephrine are used in the treatment of shock and other conditions benefited by sympathetic stimulation (asthma, allergic reactions, etc.). The catecholamines are neither pure alpha nor pure beta stimulators, but, rather, exert both alpha and beta effects. Phenylephrine has almost pure alpha activity, and isoproterenol has almost pure beta activ-

176

ARTERIOLAR VASODILATION

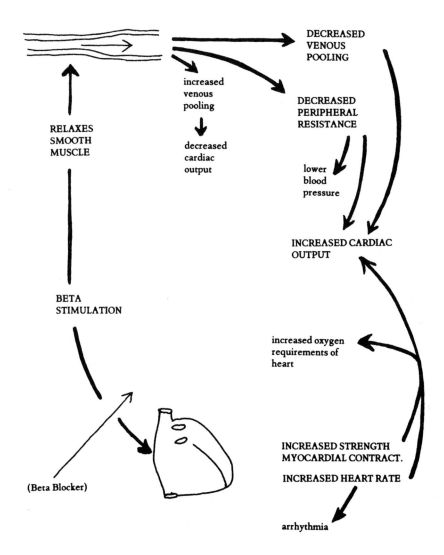

DECREASED
VENOUS
POOLING

increased
venous
pooling

DECREASED
PERIPHERAL
RESISTANCE

RELAXES
SMOOTH
MUSCLE

decreased
cardiac
output

lower
blood
pressure

INCREASED CARDIAC
OUTPUT

BETA
STIMULATION

increased oxygen
requirements of
heart

INCREASED STRENGTH
MYOCARDIAL CONTRACT.

INCREASED HEART RATE

(Beta Blocker)

arrhythmia

Figure 9.8   Beta Adrenergic Stimulation

ity. In any given situation, either alpha or beta effects may predominate, depending on many variables we understand (pH, the dosage given, the presence or absence of other catecholamines or serotonin, the presence of other drugs, a history of recent sympathetic stimulation, etc.) and many variables we don't as yet fully understand.

When given therapeutically, and when we are able to control some of the variables noted above, we can predict with a certain degree of assurance the dominant effect of these drugs.

The effects, dosage, clinical uses and complications are noted in Table 7.

In addition to the sympathetic stimulators (the catecholamines), there are other substances which nullify the effects of sympathetic stimulation. These are the adrenergic blocking agents, and are also divided into either alpha or beta according to their dominant blocking effect. The alpha adrenergic blocking agents are phenoxybenzamine (Dibenzyline) and phentolamine (Regitine). The only clinically useful beta blocker is propranolol.

The antihistamines antagonize some of the effects of the adrenergic agents, such as salivation, sweating, hyperglycemia, eosinophilia, increased oxygen consumption, central nervous system stimulation, and bronchodilatation.

Glucagon may be used to reverse the toxic effects of propranolol in an emergency. This drug has many other cardiac effects, but is not currently used in routine care.

178

DRUGS	DOSAGE	CLINICAL USES	COMPLICATIONS/OBSERVATIONS
Methoxamine (Vasoxyl) Alpha Activator	10-20 mg IM 3-10 mg IV slowly	Hypotension. Slows AV conduction & useful in supraventricular tachycardias.	May cause reflex bradycardia. Prolonged rise in blood pressure.
Phenylephrine (neosynephrine) Alpha Activator	.8 mg IV 2-5 mg SQ or IM	Similar to norepi. Powerful vasoconstrictor Slows heart rate & increases stroke volume. Useful in shock with low peripheral resistance. Useful in treatment of PAT	May cause reflex bradycardia. Do not use in hypertension. Caution in older patients and with heart block.
Dopamine (Intropin) Alpha & Beta Activator	1- 2 micrograms/ Kg/minute IV 2-10 micrograms/ Kg/minute IV 10 micrograms/ Kg/minute IV	Increases renal blood flow. Beta stimulation. Increase in CO but not HR or BP. Alpha stimulation. Blood pressure rise. Useful in shock & low cardiac output states (failure).	May cause tachyarrhythmias. Potentiated by MAO inhibitors.

Table 7.   Sympathetic Nervous System Drugs

DRUG	DOSAGE	CLINICAL USES	COMPLICATIONS/OBSERVATIONS
Epinephrine (Adrenalin) Alpha & Beta Activator	.1-.5 mg SQ 1-8 micrograms/min IV drip .25-1 mg IV push	Most potent vasopressor. Positive inotrope & chronotrope. Used in lowered CO and shock. Most useful when peripheral resistance low. Lessens AV block. Restores cardiac rhythm following arrest.	May cause ventricular tachyarrhythmias. Makes patient nervous.
Norepinephrine (Levarterenol) (Levophed) Alpha & Beta Activator	1-4 micrograms/min IV drip	Alpha premoninates at higher doses. Positive inotrope. No effect on heart rate. Most useful when peripheral resistance low.	Same.
Metaraminol (Aramine) Alpha & Beta Activator	1-3 mg IV push or IM	Releases Norepinephrine at nerve endings & no effect if norepi depleted. Positive inotrope. Useful in transient hypotension. Not effective with prolonged use. Slow onset. Ease of administration.	May cause a strong reflex vagal response & bradycardia. Duration may be prolonged. Possible ventricular irritability.

Table 7. (Cont'd)

180

DRUG	DOSAGE	CLINICAL USES	COMPLICATIONS/OBSERVATIONS
<u>Isoproterenol</u> (Isuprel) Beta Activator	1- 6 micrograms/ min. IV drip	Decreased peripheral resistance. Positive inotrope & chronotrope. Increases ventricular rate in heart block. Useful in shock with high peripheral resistance.	Ventricular arrhythmias. Hypotension.
<u>Mephentermine</u> (Wyamine) Beta Activator (mild alpha)	10-30 mg IV or IM	Peripheral action similar to Isuprel. Decreases BP, CO and coronary flow. Useful in some hypotensive states.	Same as Isuprel.
<u>Phenoxybenzamine</u> (Dibenzyline) Alpha Blocker	1 mg/Kg IV slowly (1 hr)	Blocks alpha vasoconstrictor effects. Causes vasodilatation & increased tissue perfusion. Inhibits catecholamine induced arrhythmias.	Can cause tachycardia & hypotension. Caution in use in cerebrovascular disease or renal damage.

Table 7. (Cont'd)

181

DRUG	DOSAGE	CLINICAL USES	COMPLICATIONS/OBSERVATIONS
Phentolamine (Regitine) Alpha Blocker	1- 5 mg IV 5-10 mg PO q4-6 hrs	Short acting & useful in pheochromocytoma.	Arrhythmias, esp. tachycardias.
Propranolol (Inderal) Beta Blocker	.5 mg IV test then 1 mg q3-4 min. to total of 10-15 mg.	Blocks beta cardiac affects & decreases heart rate and CO. Negative inotrope. Useful in tachyarrhythmias & dig. induced ventricular arrhythmias.	Watch for bradycardia & hypotension. Heart failure may result. Hypoglycemia & bronchospasm can be problem.
Angiotensin Direct smooth muscle constrictor	50 micrograms SQ 3-10 " /min IV	Most powerful vasopressor. Causes sodium & water retention. Useful in anaphylactic shock & overdosage of alpha blockers. Constrictor of precapillary sphincter.	Profound bradycardia & ventricular arrhythmias. Hypertension. Decreased circulating blood volume.
Atropine Parasympathetic Blocker	.5-1.0 mg IM or IV	Increases heart rate in sinus & nodal bradycardia, WPW Syn., & in 1st & 2nd degree block with bradycardia.	Contraindicated in Glaucoma, urinary retention.

Table 7. (Cont'd)

182

CHAPTER 10

TREATMENT
of
MYOCARDIAL INFARCTION

A. INTRODUCTION

Therapy for myocardial infarction may
be divided into those measures which combat
life-threatening complications and those which
relieve symptomatic distress. The latter are
useful only if they do not endanger the efficacy
of the former. Treatment should be designed
to insure adequate cardiac performance, especially during the first few days following the
acute infarct. It also should be directed toward permitting adequate scar formation in
the myocardium.

B. ENVIRONMENT

The coronary care unit is designed to
insure the appropriate surroundings necessary
for recovery. Ideally it promotes a quiet se-
rene atmosphere, but at the same time insures
the immediate availability of skilled personnel, instrumentation, and medications necessary to prevent and/or combat complications.
Constant monitoring of various cardiac functions is most important.

Since the institution of coronary care
units, the hospital mortality following an
acute myocardial infarction has dropped
from 35% to 17-20%.

C. BEDREST

At one time, it was felt that bedrest
in excess of several weeks was necessary following an infarction. Currently, it is felt

183

that early ambulation helps to prevent several complications, including thromboembolic phenomenon. A three to five day enforced bedrest seems to be adequate, if no complications intervene. Most patients will be hospitalized two to four weeks following their infarction, although we realize that adequate scar formation is not complete until at least six weeks. During the period of absolute bedrest, a Semi-Fowler's position with the feet elevated or level is desired.

D.   BOWEL FUNCTIONS

Most people subjected to absolute bedrest, even healthy people, will experience constipation. Great care must be taken with the infarct patient to insure that constipation does not occur. It is highly undesirable for a recent infarction patient to have to strain with any bowel movement. For this reason, various stool softeners and/or laxatives are routinely used in most coronary care units. Many patients cannot function normally on a bedpan. A bedside commode is indicated as soon as feasible for all infarct patients.

E.   BLADDER FUNCTIONS

For the same reason that constipation occurs with bedrest, so does urinary retention. In addition, various medication (such as atropine) will enhance the possibility of acute urinary retention. This is a complication that must be avoided. Urinary retention will cause a strong vagal response which can result in bradycardia and serious secondary arrhythmias.

It is also important to monitor the hourly urinary output. An output less than 20cc/ hour means an inadequate renal blood flow.

For the above reasons, an indwelling Foley catheter is recommended in most infarct patients.

F.   DIET

During the first two days of acute coronary care, therapy is aimed at establishing a basal metabolic state. We are attempting to allow the patient to survive with absolutely minimal bodily functions, in order to reduce the work load on the heart. Normally, the processes of ingestion, digestion, and absorption of food accounts for a large percentage of the cardiac output. For this reason, a semi-starvation and primarily liquid diet is recommended during the first 24-48 hours. Thereafter, a low cholesterol low sodium diet is allowed. If the patient is known to have a hyperlipoproteinemia, he may be placed on a proper corrective diet for this at 48 hours.

Cold food and liquids are usually forbidden, because they can cause changes on the ECG which can mimic an acute infarct pattern. Some cardiologists feel that extreme cold ingestion can cause the extension of an infarct.

G.   VITAL SIGNS

Frequent vital signs are essential when monitoring the cardiac patient. These vital signs should include the blood pressure, pulse, respiration and temperature. Urinary output should be determined hourly. The central venous or wedge pressure should likewise be done hourly (at least) during the first 48 hours. Oxygen saturation is desirable at periodic intervals during the first 2 days. If pump failure is a complication, the blood gases and pH should also be monitored.

The body weight should be recorded at least once daily. This is a sensitive indicator of fluid retention and incipient heart failure. A bed scale is the best device for doing this.

H.   CARDIAC MONITORING
(by electrocardioscope)

The primary cause of death following myocardial infarction is arrhythmia. The great success of the coronary care units has been in the early recognition and treatment of these arrhythmias – and this means constant cardiac monitoring, especially during the first 48 hours following the infarct. The minimal and maximal limit devices (for heart rate) should be set at a reasonable limit (60 and 110), and the audio alarm should never be turned off.

Several positions are used for placement of the monitor electrodes. The important consideration for electrode placement is the visibility of the P wave. The P wave can usually be best demonstrated by a placement of the leads similar to Lead V1. See Figure 10.1.

I.   MEDICATIONS

This topic has been discussed in several other chapters.

The only requirements in an uncomplicated myocardial infarction are the monitor, oxygen and an intravenous infusion line.

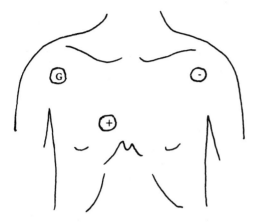

Figure 10.1   Monitor Electrodes (MCL$_1$)

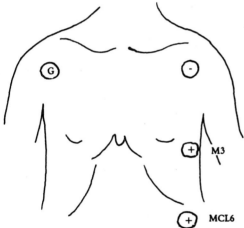

Figure 10.1a   Two Alternative Electrode Positions

187

J.   EDUCATION

Both the CCU nurse and the attending physician should take an active part in patient education. This should start in the acute phase and continue through convalescence. The patient should be taught the meaning of a heart attack and the reasonable limitations it may place on his activity and occupation. The patient and his family should receive some orientation as to the function of the CCU, and they should be prepared for his eventual transfer from the unit. It has been shown that patients who are warned beforehand of their transfer to the general medical ward do not have a rise in endogenous catecholamines, as do the patients who do not receive such advance notice. Some hospitals have CCU pamphlets which are distributed to the patient's family explaining the function and limitations of the CCU. This should also describe the reasons for visiting limitations.

The patient should also receive instructions in limiting risk factors (see Chapter 13) and the reasons why. He should also receive thorough instructions in diet therapy. The patient should be taught to be aware of symptoms of various late complications of myocardial infarction, and he should be told the rationale and importance of his discharge . medications.

The coronary patient is in a very vulnerable condition emotionally and is usually willing to accept any information or advice following his infarct. The physician and nurse should take advantage of this vulnerable period to educate the patient as much as possible.

CHAPTER 11

CARDIAC EMERGENCY
and
BASIC LIFE SUPPORT

A.   INTRODUCTION

The current standards for cardiopulmonary resuscitation are those adopted by the National Conference on Cardiopulmonary Resuscitation and Emergency Cardiac Care held in
May 1973 in Washington, D. C. This conference was co-sponsored by the American Heart
Association and the National Academy of Sci-
ences – National Research Council. The National Committee for Emergency Coronary
Care (est. in 1970) has accepted the standards
of the above conference and has promulgated
the recommendations of the conference with little change. The reader must realize that the
optimum treatment of any medical emergency
is constantly changing, and the recommendations of the above conference were quite ada-
mant in not limiting the rescuer in applying
new concepts or advances. This chapter will
deal with the current standards and recommendations of the conference.

Emergency coronary care may be best
understood as a community-wide system offer-
ing acute care to the coronary patient. The
first level of care is the emergency life support
unit which offers basic life support emergency
care. This consists primarily of cardiopulmonary resuscitation (CPR) and should be started by the first person on the scene. It must
be offered by ambulance crews, firemen, po-
lice, and emergency room personnel. This
is the first link in the chain of emergency cardiac care (ECC) and is the most important,
since only with the successful application of
basic life support care will the victim survive
for application of more advanced care.

189

In some areas of the country, the basic life support unit may have the training and equipment to apply advanced life support techniques. These emergency units may also be considered mobile life support units, in specific areas of the country. Where there is no such unit, the emergency unit will eventually find it necessary to transfer the victim to a mobile unit for transport to the next level of care, which is the acute care hospital and coronary care unit (CCU).

There is a significant difference in the capabilities of the basic and advanced life support units. This will become apparent as we describe the functions of each.

B.   BASIC LIFE SUPPORT

Basic life support is the recognition of cardiac or pulmonary (respiratory) arrest and initiating proper cardiopulmonary resuscitation until more advanced support can be started, or until transport to a facility where this can be had. It consists of the three ABC steps of CPR.

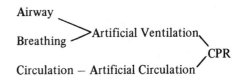

The above three steps are performed in order and as promptly as possible. Time is of the essence in effective CPR.

1.   Airway

<u>Is the victim breathing</u>? This must be determined rapidly by looking, listening, and feeling for spontaneous respiration. If the victim is not breathing, he must be ventilated. Before this can be done an adequate

airway must be available. The simplest way to achieve an airway is by the <u>held-tilt method</u>. This amounts to tilting the victim's head backwards as far as possible. This maneuver results in opening the pharynx and lifts the tongue off the back of the throat. See Figure 11.1.

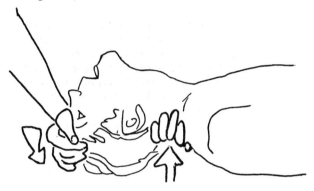

Figure 11.1   The Head-Tilt Method

The jaw thrust technique can also be used to establish an airway. This is performed by placing the fingers of both hands behind the angles of the jaw and forcing the entire jaw forward. The head is tilted backward at the same time, and the thumbs can be used to pull the mouth open. A third method is to grasp the victim's jaw with one hand by holding the mandible and lower teeth and pulling it forward, while the other hand is placed on the forehead, tilting it backwards.

In patients with head injuries or where there is a doubt of neck or cervical spine injuries, the rescuer must rely on the latter two techniques and not use the head-tilt method.

The head-tilt method is best achieved with one hand placed in back of the neck and the other on the forehead. After the proper position is achieved, it may be maintained by placing a pillow, bolster, wadded-up towel, etc. under the victim's shoulders. The head-tilt method should not be exaggerated in infants and children. Due to the extreme pliability of their tissues, the trachea (windpipe) may be collapsed by so doing.

2. Breathing

Occasionally, with the establishment of an airway, the victim will resume spontaneous respirations. If this does not occur, or if the respiratory efforts are inadequate, one must begin artificial ventilation immediately. This can be performed by various methods: mouth-to-mouth, mouth-to-nose, mouth-to-airway, or by using various ventilatory adjuncts.

Mouth-to-mouth Breathing. This is used primarily for adult resuscitation. With the head in a position to maintain an airway, the nose is pinched closed with one hand. After taking a double-sized breath, the rescuer puts his open mouth over the victim's open mouth, forming a tight seal. The rescuer then breathes into the victim's mouth with four quick double-sized breaths. After each breath, the rescuer's mouth is removed from the victim's, allowing the victim to exhale passively. The rescuer removes his mouth from the victim's by turning his head toward the victim's chest, but does not move away from the victim.

The diagnosis of ventilatory arrest, the establishment of an airway, and the four quick breaths should take no longer than twenty seconds.

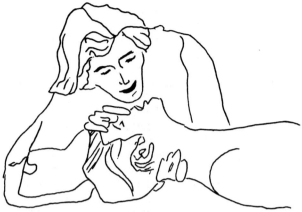

Figure 11.2   Mouth-to-Mouth Breathing

Adequate ventilation is present when
1) the victim's chest rises and falls, 2) the
rescuer feels easy transfer of his breath to
the victim, and 3) one can hear and feel the
air leaving the victim's lungs. If the above
three checks are not noted, the rescuer
must assume there is an airway obstruction
present. The victim is then rolled onto his
side and the rescuer checks the mouth and
pharynx with one or two fingers for foreign
bodies, such as loose dentures, vomitus,
etc. In doing this, a finger should be swept
back over the base of the tongue to dislodge
any solid object. Ventilation is attempted
again, and if still unsuccessful the victim is
again rolled onto his side and 2—4 sharp
blows delivered between the shoulder blades.
These two procedures are repeated until an
effective airway is established.

In performing the various maneuvers
to relieve airway obstruction, great care
must be taken while turning the unconscious
patient to protect a potentially injured

spine. The newest method recommended by the American Heart Association is designed to do just that.

Assume the victim is found lying on his abdomen. The rescuer first "shakes and shouts" to determine if the victim is unconscious. If the victim is unresponsive, he must be moved onto his back. The rescuer kneels at either side of the victim. This may be done in a full kneeling position (with both knees on the ground) or a half-kneel (with the leg nearest the victim's head in a squat position). The victim's near arm is then raised over his head and the far arm brought down to his side. The rescuer's arm nearest the victim's feet is used to stabilize the victim's spine and move the victim toward the rescuer. Constant pressure is maintained by the rescuer's elbow on the victim's far pelvis, while the same hand grasps the victim's far shoulder. The victim's far arm lies on top of the rescuer's arm. The head is stabilized by a firm grasp at the base of the skull by the rescuer's free hand. As the turning is accomplished, the victim's head will rest on his up-stretched arm. Figure 11.3

After the victim has been turned onto his back, his head is extended, and he is examined for spontaneous breathing. The rescuer's ear is placed directly over the victim's mouth, while he is looking at the victim's chest. In this position, he can LOOK at the victim's chest for a rise and fall, LISTEN for respiratory sounds, and FEEL the warm expired air from the victim's mouth. A full ten seconds should be allowed for this evaluation.

If there is no spontaneous breathing, artificial ventilation is attempted with four quick ventilations. If the three criteria for adequate ventilation are not met, the triple airway maneuver is performed. This con-

194

sists of 1) displacing the jaw forward by exerting pressure on both angles of the jaw,
2) tilting the head backward (more than
has already been done), and 3) opening the
mouth. The mouth is opened by using the
fleshy part of both thumbs.

Ventilation is again attempted, and if
still unsuccessful, it must be assumed that
an airway obstruction is present. The victim
must then be turned onto his far side in the
following manner: the victim's far arm is
placed over his head and the near arm to his
side. The rescuer's arm nearest the victim's
feet is again used to both stabilize the spine
and turn the victim. The bent elbow is placed
in back of the near side of the victim's pelvis
and the same hand on the near shoulder. The
free hand is again used to stabilize the head
as it rolls up onto the victim's up-stretched
arm. When the victim is on his side, the rescuer's leg nearest the head is brought up to
support the head, allowing free use of the
hand that was supporting the head. Using
either (or both) hands, the victim's mouth is
opened, and the back of the tongue swept
clean of foreign bodies. The mouth can be
opened by use of the scissors technique, using the fleshy part of the fingers only.
Figures 11.5 and 11.6.

After the mouth has been cleaned out,
the head is again grasped, and the victim
rolled onto his back while continued stabilization of the trunk and spine is done with
the arm nearest the victim's feet. The head
is extended and ventilation again attempted.
If still unsuccessful, the victim must be
turned toward the rescuer. The victim's
arms are reversed in position, the head stabilized, and the turn accomplished by the
rescuer's same arm applied this time to the
far side of the victim (as when turning the
victim from a face-down position). When the

victim is on his side, his head can again be supported by the rescuer's leg. Either hand can be used to deliver two to four sharp blows between the shoulder blades.

While the head is stabilized with the free hand, the victim is rolled onto his back again, his head extended, and ventilation attempted. If still unsuccessful, the entire maneuver is repeated--turn away to clear mouth and turn toward to deliver blows.

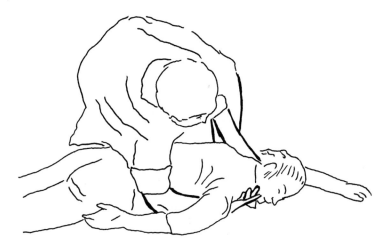

Figure 11.3 Turning Victim from Prone
Position

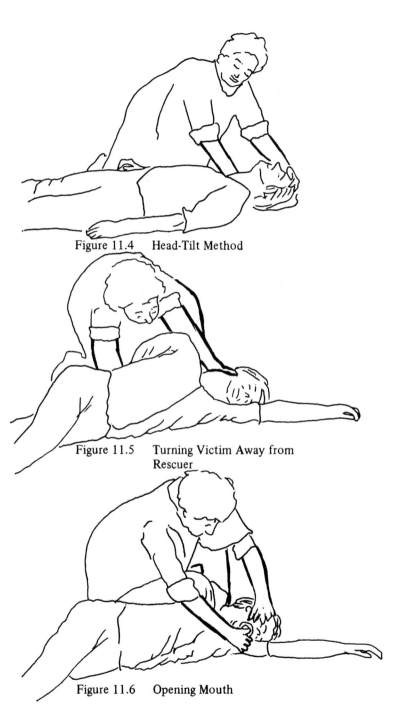

Figure 11.4   Head-Tilt Method

Figure 11.5   Turning Victim Away from
Rescuer

Figure 11.6   Opening Mouth

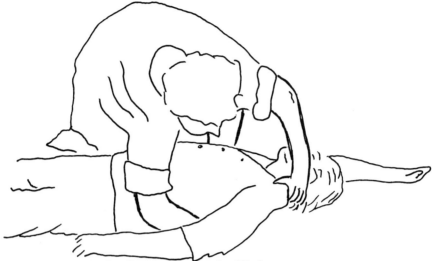

Figure 11.7   Position for Turning Victim
Toward Rescuer

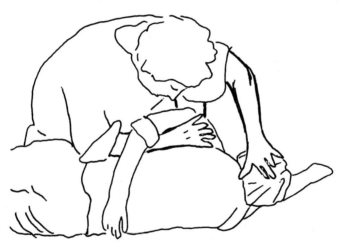

Figure 11.8   Position for Blows to Back

When the airway is established, the rescuer inflates the victim's lungs four times in quick succession (using double breaths), and then gives a full inflation every five seconds (12/minute). This is the procedure when there are two or more rescuers. The one rescuer technique is different and will be discussed later. A convenient cadence to use during the above is to the count of "one-thousand and one, one-thousand and two," etc. On the count of "one-thousand and three" the rescuer prepares for the inflation, and on the count of "one-thousand and five" inflates the victim's lungs. This is called the 1 to 5 technique and is used with two or more rescuers only. (The 2 to 15 technique is used with one rescuer.) In infants and children, the inflation rate is every three seconds, or a minimum of twenty per minute. In infants, it is most convenient to place the rescuer's mouth over the mouth and nose of the victim. The inflation pressure necessary for infant ventilation is much less than in an adult. The rescuer may judge the proper amount of pressure by watching for the rise and fall of the chest during ventilation. The smallest amount of pressure to give this rise and fall should be used.

There are several variations in ventilatory techniques which can be used. The mouth-to-nose technique is more aesthetic to some people and is absolutely necessary if an injury to the victim's mouth prevents adequate seal for the mouth-to-mouth technique. The mouth-to-stoma technique is required in patients with a tracheostomy. The rate and ratio of ventilation is the same with these variations.

Ventilatory adjuncts are devices which aid in the maintenance of an airway or aid in the ready delivery of artificial ventilation. The basic life support rescuer is expected to be able to use a number of these devices.

Airway adjuncts are rubber or plastic
devices to insure the maintenance of the airway once it has been established by the steps
noted above. These are called oropharyngeal
airways and are available in a number of
makes and styles. See Figure 11.9.

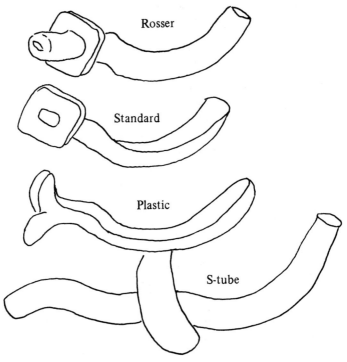

Figure 11.9   Artificial Airways

They all have in common an oral curve
which conforms to the soft tissues of the
floor of the mouth, and keeps the tongue depressed to allow air to the back of the throat.
These should be used whenever a bag-valve-
mask system is used or when a breathing device with mask is used. They should only be
used on unconscious patients, and they
should be inserted with some care to prevent
airway obstruction. They should be fitted
to the patient, and sizes for infants and chil-

dren should be available. S-tubes, although aesthetically more pleasing, have numerous shortcomings which make them less desirable than the standard oropharyngeal airway. There is much difficulty maintaining a tight seal around the flange of the S-tube.

These devices are all inserted in the same way. If possible they should be lubricated before insertion with a standard surgical lubricant or water. During insertion, the head and neck of the victim must be maintained in a position for proper airway, and artificial ventilation should not be interrupted for more than five seconds. Working from the head of the patient, the tip of the airway is directed into the mouth with the curve pointed toward the palate (top of the mouth), while the other hand holds the mouth open by grasping the lower jaw and pulling it forward and downward. As insertion continues, an obstruction will be met when the airway hits the back of the throat (posterior soft palate or posterior pharynx). The airway is gently rotated so that the tip now points in the direction of the trachea and is carefully advanced until the flange is flush with the lips. The mouth is then closed, and a clear plastic breathing mask applied, if one is using the straight airway. If the S-tube is used, the seal at the flange is checked and mouth-to-tube ventilation commenced. In either case, ventilation is started immediately and the adequacy of the airway checked by watching the victim's chest and listening for the escape of air during exhalation.

Breathing or ventilatory adjuncts are devices to aid artificial ventilation after the airway has been established. They can be used only after an artificial airway has been inserted. Masks, if used, should be of clear plastic and be available in a variety of sizes.

The fit and seal must be carefully checked with each victim. Bellows devices are not recommended because they are ineffectual in providing adequate ventilation. Bag-valve-mask devices are effective when used by personnel trained in their use and are most effective when used in conjunction with an endotracheal tube. The "Air-Viva" device is made specifically for emergency bag-valve-mask resuscitation and works quite well.

Positive pressure breathing devices are quite useful after a properly functioning airway is established. These devices can be triggered manually to provide artificial ventilation or can be set to offer ventilatory assistance only (triggered by the patient's own respiratory efforts). These should not be used in infants and children unless the pressure has been set specifically for this purpose. These devices must be used with an oxygen source, and some familiarity with the use of medical oxygen is necessary. The "Elder Demand Valve" and the "Blount Demand Valve" are two approved and commonly used positive pressure breathing devices. Both can be used with a mask or with an endotracheal tube.

The Conference has established criteria and standards for all these adjuncts and the reader is referred to the full Conference report for a discussion of these.

A nasal cannula is a device of polyethylene tubing which allows the delivery of oxygen at 30-35% to a patient who is breathing spontaneously. It must be connected to a flow meter to regulate the amount of oxygen delivered and to a humidifier bottle to moisten the oxygen gas. It is very simply installed by placing the two nasal tips in the nostrils and securing the whole device with an elastic strap around the head.

Oxygen may also be delivered at 60% concentration by the use of a plastic face mask, which is held in place by an elastic strap. A flow meter and humidifier must also be used. This is to be used only after the patient is breathing spontaneously.

When using oxygen for any purpose, certain precautions must be taken. Oxygen is an extremely explosive gas and care should be taken that all cigarettes, matches, and other sources of detonation are kept far away. Oxygen stored in cylinders is under great pressure and it must be reduced before delivery to the patient. Most medical oxygen cylinders are equipped with a combination regulator-reduction valve which reduces the pressure to the flow meter to 50PSI. Some of these valves are attached to the cylinder contents gauge. After the gas passes through the reduction valve it goes to the flow meter where the amount of oxygen delivered to the patient is determined. The proper amount when using the nasal cannula or plastic mask is 2-6L/min. A larger amount is required with the positive pressure devices.

Pure oxygen has a very drying effect on the mucosa of the respiratory tract. For this reason, it must be humidified before it reaches the patient. Humidifier bottles are used for this purpose, and are filled with sterile distilled water.

When oxygen is used from a hospital wall outlet, a reduction valve is not necessary, but a flow meter and humidifier bottle are.

It should be remembered that the faster the oxygen flow, the less humidified the oxygen becomes.

During artificial ventilation it is common for some of the instilled air to get into

the stomach, and it will eventually cause
gastric distention. Gross distention can
cause pressure on the diaphragm and prevent
adequate cardiac functions. This can be re-
lieved by exerting moderate pressure over the
stomach, forcing the air out the mouth.
When this is done, the victim's head should
be turned to the side to prevent aspiration
of vomitus.

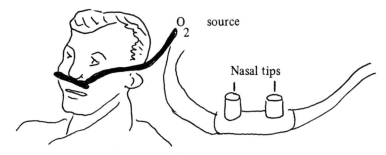

Figure 11.10   Nasal cannula

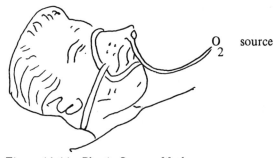

Figure 11.11   Plastic Oxygen Mask

3. Circulation

While the rescuer is manipulating the
head and neck during airway and breathing
procedures, the carotid pulse may be felt.
It should specifically be checked after the
first four ventilations. If it is absent, artificial circulation should be started as soon as

204

possible. The carotid pulse can be checked
by first feeling the thyroid cartilage (larynx
or voice box) and then sliding the fingers
down the sides of the cartilage to the groove
between the trachea (windpipe) and the
sternocleidomastoid muscle. Gentle pressure
in this area should discover the pulse, if it is
present.

   The heart lies in the lower mediastinum
in the midline between the vertebral column
and the sternum (breast bone). Pressure on
the lower half of the sternum of sufficient
weight, will compress the sternum and force
blood out of the ventricles. In adults, the
weight necessary to do this is 80-120 lbs.
This is the rationale of cardiac compression.
See Figure 11.12.

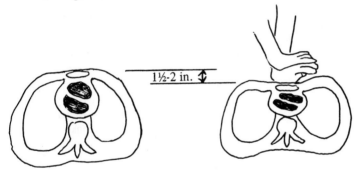

1½-2 in.

Figure 11.12   Cardiac Compression in
                        Adults.

   Cardiac compression should not be attempted unless the victim is lying on a firm
support. The average bed is not a firm support, and before cardiac compression is
started, a back support should be put into
place or the victim placed on the floor or
ground.

205

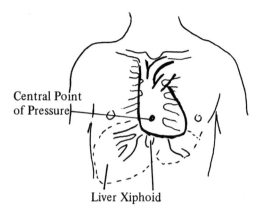

Central Point
of Pressure

Liver Xiphoid

Figure 11.13   Position for hand

The butt of one hand is placed over the lower half of the sternum, one inch above the xiphoid process, and the other hand on top of the first. Care should be exercised not to place the hands over the xiphoid process. The rescuer should position himself at the victim's side, or if done in a bed, while standing on a short lift. Sufficient pressure should be used to compress the sternum 1½ to 2 inches, while care is taken that the fingers of the lower hand do not touch the chest. The compressions should be regular, smooth, and uninterrupted at a rate of 60/minute (with two or more rescuers. The one rescuer technique will be described later). The proper cadence is one compression to each count as described above under Breathing. All pressure should be removed between compressions, but without removing the hands from the chest. This is to allow adequate venous filling of the heart between compressions.

The above technique must be modified for infants and children. The amount of compression should obviously be less than in an

adult, and the rate of compression is faster —
100 per minute. An infant can be resuscitat-
ed by one person during transport. In small
infants, the rescuer's hand can be placed
around the entire chest and compress the
precordium between the thumb and middle
finger. One rescuer ratio is 5:1.

It has been shown that external cardiac
compression done properly can produce palpable peripheral pulses, and this can be
checked for during resuscitation. This is done
by using either the carotid or femoral artery
pulsations, but should be done only if there
are two or more rescuers. A single rescuer
should never stop resuscitory efforts to check
the pulse, but rather wait for signs of spontaneous revival. It should also be mentioned
that a palpable pulse means only that the
blood is circulating, and does not mean that
it is oxygenated. Equal effort must be spent
on breathing as on cardiac compression.

There are several conditions in which
external cardiac compression will not prove
effective. As mentioned above, the efficacy
of external cardiac compression depends on
the midline position of the heart (between
the sternum and the vertebral column). If
for any reason the heart is not in the midline, external cardiac compression will not
result in effective blood flow, and internal
cardiac compression must be instituted.
This procedure will be discussed in a later
section. Chest wall injuries or other conditions resulting in a tension pneumothorax
(where the heart is displaced to one side or
the other) make external cardiac compression
ineffective. These conditions usually require
management with more sophisticated equipment and skills, than found in the basic life
support team. Even the diagnosis of these
conditions requires equipment not found

in the emergency team. Resuscitation will not be effective in many patients suffering severe stroke and in accident victims with injuries so severe as to be incompatible with life.

4. One Rescuer Technique

The ideal life support technique is with a minimum of two rescuers: one to ventilate and the other to attend to cardiac compression. A third rescuer is useful to check peripheral pulses and to relieve the other two. However, in many situations, there is only one rescuer available for CPR. In this situation, the above procedures must obviously be modified. It is currently recommended that the rescuer use the 15:2 technique. After an airway has been established and four quick double breaths given the victim, the rescuer compresses the precordium 15 times at the rate of 80/minute ("One and two and three and . . .") then rapidly changes position to give the victim two double-sized ventilations within six seconds, and then back to the chest for 15 more compressions. See Figure 11.15.

The two rescuer technique has been described and is illustrated in Figure 11.14.

5. Precordial Thump

In a witnessed cardiac arrest or in other situations where an arrest is suspected and there has been a very short time since the onset of the arrest and resuscitory efforts, a precordial thump is worth while

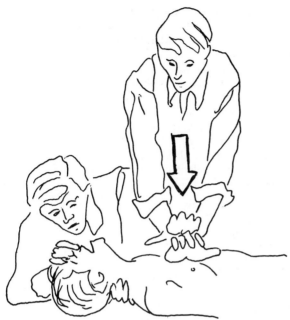

Figure 11.14 Two Rescuer Technique

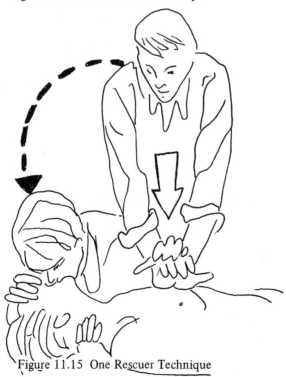

Figure 11.15 One Rescuer Technique

trying. This is usually true in patients who are being monitored in the coronary care unit. A precordial thump is a sharp blow delivered with the fleshy side of the fist to the midsternum of the victim from a distance of 8 to 12 inches. This blow delivers a measurable electric charge to the precordium and may convert a fibrillation or asystole to a regular rhythm, if done so within one minute of the arrest. No time should be wasted on the precordial thump if more than one minute has elapsed, and it should not be performed on children.

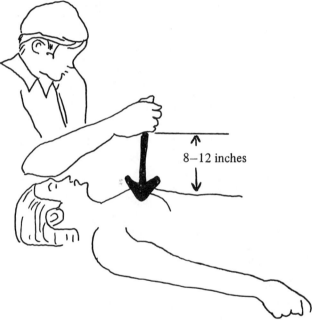

8–12 inches

Figure 11.16 The Precordial Thump

The procedure for a witnessed arrest is to open the airway and palpate the carotid pulse at the same time. If it is not present, a precordial thump is delivered and compression started.

A similar technique is used in the monitored patient with ventricular fibrillation, ventricular tachycardia, or asystole. The protocol for such a patient is as follows:

1.   Precordial thump.
2.   Check the monitor for rhythm and the carotid pulse.
3.   If ventricular tachycardia is present and there is no pulse, or if ventricular fibrillation is present, countershock.
4.   If pulse is absent, check airway and start artificial ventilation with four quick inflations.
5.   Check carotid pulse again.
6.   If pulse still absent, start CPR and summon life support team.

6.   Complications of CPR

Gastric distention has already been mentioned and is quite common, especially in children. Rib fractures and costochondral separations are also quite common, especially in older patients. These are acceptable complications. The liver may be lacerated by too vigorous compression of the sternum or by placing the hands too near the xiphoid. Internal injury can only be caused by the wrong application of the hand position. If done properly, internal injury is not necessary, although it is sometimes inevitable in older patients or in patients with underlying medical problems.

The rescuer must also consider the fact that the inevitable complication of a victim in a condition of extremis is death, and that any minor injury sustained during efforts to prevent this ultimate complication is acceptable. The author was once told by

211

a much older and wiser clinician that CPR done properly always resulted in a few rib fractures. Although this may seem a little radical, especially in younger patients, the idea is still valid.

One must also mention a complication to the rescuer. If the victim has an upper or lower respiratory infection, the rescuer performing artificial ventilation may also be infected.

7.   Evaluating CPR

The carotid or femoral pulse can be used to evaluate the effectiveness of cardiac compression. Ventilation can be evaluated by the pupillary reflex. When the pupils are widely dilated and do not react to light by constricting, serious brain damage has occurred. If the pupils are widely dilated but do react to light, brain damage has not yet occurred, but the brain is not receiving adequate oxygen. It should be recognized that in older people, the pupillary reflex may be very weak or absent. Similar effects are seen with certain drugs, such as narcotics. When checking for the pupillary reflex, the rescuer should also check for artificial eyes and contact lenses.

8.   Terminating CPR

Basic life support should be continued until:

1.   Adequate breathing and circulation have been resumed by the victim.
2.   Another responsible rescuer has taken over.
3.   A physician assumes responsibility.
4.   The victim is transferred to trained medical or paramedical personnel.

212

5. The rescuer can no longer continue. The rescuer should not continue to the point of exhaustion.

6. The coroner or a physician pronounces the patient dead.

9. Who Does CPR?

Basic life support is a learned skill in which, by law, all law enforcement officers, firemen, and ambulance attendants must be proficient. It is also strongly recommended by the Conference that all RNs, LVNs, and physicians be proficient at CPR and be certified for continued proficiency on a six-month or yearly basis.

C. ADVANCED LIFE SUPPORT

Advanced life support connotes basic life support plus more advanced equipment, techniques, and skills. Advanced life support should be available in every emergency room and CCU in the country. It includes:

1. Basic life support and use of basic adjuncts.

2. The use of advanced adjunctive equipment and special techniques, such as endotracheal intubation and open chest cardiac compression.

3. Cardiac monitoring.

4. ' Defibrillation.

5. Initiation and maintenance of intravenous fluids.

6. Definitive therapy for acidosis and arrhythmias.

7. Stabilization of the patient.

1. Airway and Ventilation Adjuncts

Numerous adjuncts are available for airway maintenance and ventilatory assistance. Oxygen is the most commonly used of all adjuncts in CPR and with good reason. The brain and heart have a very low tolerance to hypoxia, and any increase in the blood oxygen content will improve the chance of these two organs to survive.

Oropharyngeal airways, masks, and positive pressure breathing devices were discussed in the section on basic life support. It is axiomatic that the advanced life support team is proficient in the use of these devices.

The esophageal obturator airway is a relatively new device which obstructs the esophagus while allowing all inflated air to go into the trachea and lungs. It can be inserted blindly, but the inherent dangers to the esophagus limit its usefulness to properly trained personnel.

Endotracheal intubation is a well established means of delivering artificial ventilation. When used with a cuffed tube, there is little or no danger of aspiration of gastric contents or of gastric dilitation. However, these devices must never be inserted by one who is inexperienced in their use, and this limits their usefulness. Indications for endotracheal intubation are:

    1.   Cardiac arrest.
    2.   Respiratory arrest.
    3.   Inability of the rescuer to ventilate the victim by conventional means.
    4.   Deep coma.
    5.   Need for prolonged artificial ventilation.

These tubes should be available in a variety of sizes with uncuffed tubes for infants and children. During insertion of these tubes, CPR should not be interrupted for longer than five seconds at a time.

Suction devices should be available for tracheal aspiration and must provide sufficient air-flow for this purpose. These can be either the permanently installed or portable variety, but must be available at the head of the patient. Accessory equipment must be easily cleaned and decontaminated and should be non-kinking and sterile. The amount of suction should be controlled. Various size suction catheters should be available.

Nasogastric tubes should be available for gastric decompression.

2.   Circulation Adjuncts

Bedboards or spine boards are an absolute necessity for CPR, and should be placed under the victim before any cardiac compression takes place. They should be covered by a slick material or have a slick finish for sliding under the patient.

Manual chest compressors are useful in continuing external cardiac compression after initial CPR has been started. Automatic compressors provide uninterrupted cardiac compression in an effective way. Both of these devices are designed to be installed on the patient in a minimum period of time with little interruption of life support measures. The automatic devices are heavy and rather cumbersome and have many hazards. They must be monitored closely when in use and are still under investigation.

Internal cardiac compression involves the opening of the chest and the manual compression of the heart with the rescuer's hand. This technique should only be used when it is the only alternative to certain death, as in cardiac tamponade, and then only by a physician experienced in the technique, and under controlled circumstances.

215

3.   Cardiac Monitoring

As soon as possible, the patient's cardiac rhythm must be monitored. This should not however, interrupt the basic life support measures. The most convenient method of determining the initial cardiac rhythm is with the monitor-defibrillator device in which the paddles are also the monitor electrodes.

Advanced life support personnel must be able to recognize the following electrocardiographic arrhythmias:

1.   Asystole.
2.   Bradycardia (rate less than 60).
3.   Supraventricular and ventricular rhythms.
4.   PVCs.
5.   Ventricular tachycardia.
6.   Ventricular fibrillation.
7.   AV blocks.
8.   Atrial fibrillation and flutter.

Advanced life support personnel must be knowledgeable of the complications of the above arrhythmias, which arrhythmias are life threatening and the therapy of each.

4.   Defibrillation

Defibrillation causes a simultaneous depolarization of all the myocardium which may be followed by a regular rhythm. This is the immediate treatment for ventricular fibrillation and ventricular tachycardia with no peripheral pulse. It is of no use in asystole. Defibrillation causes no permanent damage to the heart and can thusly be used in arrest before the monitor leads have been put in place, on the chance that ventricular fibrillation is present. This is not recommended on children. The usual shock of 300-400 Watt seconds is usually adequate although much smaller shocks may work.

Defibrillation can be dangerous to the personnel of the life support team. The bed or cart on which it is done, should be grounded and all personnel must stand clear of the patient and bed during the procedure. CPR should not be interrupted for longer than five seconds if defibrillation is not successful. The proper placement of the defibrillator paddles is shown in Figure 11.17.

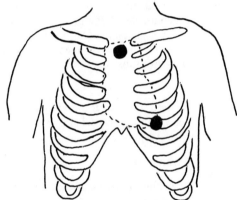

Figure 11.17   Defibrillator Paddle Placement. ●

Treatment of acidosis and hypoxemia is sometimes necessary before defibrillation or CPR is effective.

5.   Intravenous Lifeline

This is quite essential for the treatment of arrhythmias, acidosis, or shock — all the immediate complications of acute myocardial infarction — and should be started as soon as possible after basic life support has been initiated. The percutaneous needle or catheter must be a large bore one.

217

6.   Drug Therapy

Most drug therapy in the CPR patient is by the intravenous route. Occasionally intracardiac epinephrine is used, but should be done so only by a physician experienced in this method and only when an IV has not been started. Epinephrine and lidocaine are effective when instilled directly into the tracheobronchial tree. Lidocaine and atropine are effective for arrhythmia control when given by the intramuscular route, but this is not recommended due to the unknown nature of the peripheral circulation in an arrest patient. Intramuscular injection will also interfere with subsequent serum CPK determination.

Drugs used in the CPR patient have been divided into the essential and useful categories.

Essential Drugs

Sodium Bicarbonate
Epinephrine
Atropine Sulfate
Lidocaine
Morphine Sulfate
Calcium Chloride
Oxygen

1. Sodium Bicarbonate is essential in the treatment of metabolic acidosis. It is given in the dose of 1mEq/kg by either bolus or continuous IV drip. It is given every 10 minutes of arrest until effective circulation is re-established. After the second dose and before the third dose is given, a blood pH, blood gases, and serum sodium should be done by the laboratory. This is so the clinician may be aware of the possible onset of metabolic alkalosis or hyperosmolality from excessive medication. Bicarbonate is marketed in prefilled syringes and ampoules of 44.6 and 50 mEq.

2. Epinephrine is given every five
minutes during resuscitation in the dose of
.5cc or 1:1000 diluted in 10cc of sterile
water or saline, or 5cc of 1:10,000 solution.
The latter is marketed in prefilled syringes.
Epinephrine has a positive inotropic effect,
increases perfusion pressure, and lowers the
defibrillation threshold.

3. Atropine sulfate is given intravenously for bradycardia with escape PVCs
or hypotension in the dose of .5mg every
five minutes until a total dose of 2mg has
been given or the heart rate increases to 60
or more. Some clinicians prefer an initial
dose of 1mg.

4. Lidocaine increases the fibrillation threshold by depressing automaticity
of the myocardium, and by the same mechanism abolishes PVCs. It should not be
given if complete heart block is present, unless a pacemaker has already been inserted.
It is usually given as a bolus of 50-100mg
followed by an IV drip of 1-4mg/minute.
It is available in prefilled syringes.

5. Morphine sulfate is not indicated
in CPR but is quite useful in later therapy of
acute myocardial infarction or pulmonary
edema. The respiratory depression seen with
the normal therapeutic dose of 12-15mg can
be avoided by slow intravenous injections of
3-4.5mg at 5 to 30 minute intervals.

6. Calcium chloride is useful in complete cardiovascular collapse by restoring an
electrical rhythm in asystole and by enhancing defibrillation. It is given in doses of
2.5-5cc of the 10% solution in an IV bolus.
Calcium gluconate is given in doses of 10cc
of the 10% solution. Calcium must be given
with care with concomitant digitalis therapy
and should not be given at the same time as
bicarbonate.

Useful Drugs

Vasoactive drugs
  Levarterenol (Levophed)
  Metaraminol (Aramine)
  Dopamine
  Isoproterenol   (Isuprel)
  Propranolol   (Inderal)
  Corticosteroids

1. Vasoactive drugs are not indicated in every patient with acute MI nor even with every CPR patient. The use of these compounds in shock or hypotension during and after CPR is not unanimous among cardiovascular authorities. Their use runs the risk of further decrease in cerebral, coronary and renal blood flow. One must weigh the potential advantages of their use against the potential dangers. Dopamine promises to be the most useful and least dangerous of the group.

2. Isoproterenol has been discussed in an earlier chapter. Its use in shock following acute MI can result in further extension of the infarct, and accordingly its use in this syndrome must be discouraged. However, it is quite useful in other forms of shock where there is a high peripheral resistance. It increases the heart rate, is a positive inotrope, and reduces the peripheral resistance. It is given in doses of 2-20 micrograms/minute by IV drip.

3. Propranolol is useful in the treatment of bradycardia with complete heart block. It must be used with caution in patients with heart failure or asthma. It is given in a dose of 1mg IV and repeated to a total of 3mg.

4. Corticosteroids. Much controversy has surrounded the use of these compounds in the past. It is currently felt that

220

their use in shock is definitely beneficial. The synthetic steroids, methylprednisolone or dexamethasone, are recommended.

7. Stabilization

Stabilization for transport to a life support unit is generally not done in the field, although it is recognized that such an approach could save many lives each year. This would involve maintaining effective ventilation, effective circulation, a stable cardiac rhythm with the use of drugs, a working monitor, an intravenous lifeline and communications for consultation with a continuing care facility, as well as telemetry.

8. Termination of Life Support

This decision is a medical one and depends on considerations which have already been discussed. A reasonable approach to termination of life support is to do so if the pupils have remained fixed and dilated for 15-30 minutes, or if there has been no sign of ventricular activity on the monitor for 10 minutes. This approach can be modified in children or under conditions of hypothermia.

D   LIFE SUPPORT UNITS

Life support units can be either basic or advanced. Basic life support units are found at all patient care stations in hospitals, medical and dental offices, factories, public office buildings, schools, etc. Advanced life support units are presumed to be found in all emergency rooms and coronary care units. Certain field units and ambulance operations also offer advanced life support.

Life support units should be offered in all public places where large numbers of people congregate — sports arenas, convention centers, stadiums, auditoriums, large industrial plants, office building complexes, major transportation terminals and commercial airlines.

Physicians and nurses manning advanced life support units must be qualified and proficient in the techniques noted above and should be recertified yearly for this proficiency.

There should also be a clear written policy that defines the areas of responsibility. Continued educational programs for life support unit personnel are strongly recommended, and are absolutely required to maintain the level of proficiency required with newer techniques and methods.

The Conference has established a list of necessary drugs and equipment needed to offer advanced life support. The reader is referred to the report.

E   THE TEAM

There is no phase of medicine that requires the team approach more than in the application of basic and advanced life support. Each member of the life support team must have his duties precisely defined. Each member must also be familiar with the duties of the other members and be able to assume these duties in their absence. Every member of the team must be able to start basic life support while the rest of the team is summoned. As each member arrives, he must be able to assume the job most critically needed at the time. When the entire team is present, each member can then perform his own task. This type of team effort is not

something that is learned from a book like
this. It comes with practice and more practice.

Each team should have periodic drills
in both basic and advanced life support. A
responsible observer should be present to
evaluate the drill. Each drill should be followed immediately by a critique period,
during which each member may give his
impressions of the drill and all members reflect on the impressions of the observer.

Certain precautions may be helpful to
the team. 1) Do not panic. Panic and hys-
teria are contagious and have no place on a
life support team. The job is done best by
a quiet, efficient team, with each member
doing his job in an undisturbed and undis-
turbing way. 2) After life support has begun and the team is functioning properly,
do not hurry. The old adage "Haste makes
waste" is no more true than in the functioning of a life support team. 3) Keep unnecessary personnel away. The ideal team consists of five of six members. Additional
people get in the way and slow down an
otherwise efficient operation. 4) Each
team must have a designated leader. Each
member of the team must follow the direction of the leader, even if he or she seems
to be in variance with standard procedures.
Remember that each patient is different,
and what might be applicable to most may
not be applicable to this one. In most situations, the physician member of the team
is the leader, but this may not necessarily
be true. In teaching institutions, the CCU
nurse may well be the team leader, even
when a physician is present. Until the physician arrives, the RN is the leader, and until she arrives, the LVN is the leader.

223

The members of the life support team should assume the following job descriptions:

1. Maintain airway and breathing.
2. Circulation (cardiac compression).
3. Starting and maintenance of IV.
4. Circulating nurse.
5. Recorder and time keeper.
6. Traffic control.

If specialized personnel arrive to help (such as a ventilation therapist), the leader may indicate that the member performing that function move to a different function or be excused altogether. Jobs 1. and 2. are physically exhausting and should be rotated among other members of the team.

At the end of each life support episode, a Life Support Report Form should be completed. This Form should describe everything that was done and the time recorded. It should also list the members present and their time of arrival. Of course, the patient's chart must receive similar notations. The information on the Form should also include any complications that were encountered and the way in which they were managed, types of arrhythmias noted and their management, and whether the efforts of the team were successful or unsuccessful. These forms should be kept separate from the patient's chart. At regular intervals, the forms collected in this way should be reviewed by the life support team and by the CCU committee. In this way, the team may see where it has been successful and also where it has been unsuccessful, and perhaps patterns can be picked up to explain the latter. This amounts to a Life Support Audit.

F. CONCLUSION

Everyone involved in direct patient care in a hospital should be able to recognize the need for, and be able to initiate basic life support procedures. This means not only physicians and nurses, but also therapists and nursing assistants. In smaller hospitals where a minimum of medical personnel may be on hand at certain times, other personnel should participate in CPR training — such as ward clerks, laboratory and X-ray technicians, housekeeping staff, etc. Personnel should be certified for adequacy of life support training and recertified at appropriate intervals — usually not to exceed one year.

Advanced life support should be offered in every emergency room and CCU-ICU of every acute care hospital. This is mainly the responsibility of physicians, nurses, and ancillary personnel, such as inhalation therapists. In addition, it is recommended that advanced life support responsibility be shared with mobile life support units and that proper training and certification be made available for this. Implementation of mobile life support units requires a communications system between them and the CCU. This type of mobile life support unit can currently be found in a few major metropolitan areas.

CHAPTER 12

THE CORONARY CARE UNIT

A.   HISTORY

The coronary care unit is just over ten years old. One of the first published reports of a CCU was from New York Hospital-Cornell Medical Center in May 1968. This paper described the evolution of their four-bed unit from its inception in January 1965 to January 1967.

The unit had all the equipment we currently use in a CCU, and the nursing staff was trained in the recognition of arrhythmias. The treatment of arrhythmias was left up to the discretion of the house staff assigned to the CCU, and there was a wide variety of approaches to the treatment of arrhythmias as to the medication used and the time it was given. After the first 100 cases had been treated in the CCU, a comparison was made of 100 cardiac patients treated during the same period of time on the general medical wards. It was discouraging to find that the statistics were exactly the same. The CCU had not affected the mortality rate at all.

As a result of the above findings, a more aggressive and organized approach to the treatment of arrhythmias was adopted. Routine protocol was established for the use of antiarrhythmic drugs and cardioversion. Speed of application of definitive measures was stressed. The CCU nurses were given additional training in advanced life support and were given the responsibility of initiating these measures, when indicated (including drug administration, defibrillation, and cardiac pacing). The statistical results following the institution of these new measures was startling. In the absence of shock, the mortality rate was reduced from 26% to 7%. When shock was present, it was reduced from 85% to 69%. Similar results have been obtained across the country.

The CCU is now a routine established procedure for the treatment of acute myocardial infarctions. The rationale for the CCU is the prompt recognition and treatment of life threatening arrhythmias, and the early diagnosis and treatment of the other complications of myocardial infarction (heart failure), shock, and surgical complications). The need and function of the CCU is now well established. Let us now consider the many factors that make up a true CCU.

B.   PHYSICAL DESIGN

The size of the CCU depends on the number of annual admissions and the ability of the hospital to maintain staffing. In very small hospitals, a one-bed private room (meeting all the other requirements of a CCU) is adequate. In some hospitals, the CCU may be combined with the intensive care unit (ICU). In this case, great care must be taken to insure the integrity and function of each unit. The smallest unit which is economically feasible, as an independent unit, is the four-bed unit. A six-bed unit is even more economical, since it requires no additional staffing.

The CCU may be incorporated into an already-existent facility or be added to the plans of a new facility. In any case, it should be somewhat away from the major traffic flow of the facility, but within close proximity to the emergency room, for prompt transport of cardiac admissions.

228

Each bed on the unit should be separate from the other beds, in order to reduce unnecessary psychological trauma. This is best achieved by having private rooms available. Each room should have monitoring and resuscitation equipment. Because of the necessity of close surveillance, each bed should be within full view of the nursing module. This also allays patient anxiety of "being alone". The minimum floor space allowable for each bed is determined by Public Health Standards.

The CCU bed-module should be as tranquil as possible, since this seems to have a suppressant effect on arrhythmias. Acoustical ceilings and flooring are recommended. A radio, clock, and calendar are also recommended to allay patient anxiety. Adequate lighting is essential, and bedside suction and oxygen outlets are a necessity. Ideally, the CCU should be functionally independent from the rest of the facility. This means a separate nurses' station (within view of each bed), a work area, supply area, medication area, and staff lavatory. When the CCU is combined with the ICU, additional facilities may be needed.

Proper temperature and humidity control are necessary, and this requires air-conditioning. The area should be electrically independent from the rest of the facility, and alternate emergency power is a must. Routine electronic maintenance is necessary to insure proper grounding of all equipment (see section on Electrical Hazards in this Chapter).

C.   EQUIPMENT

Each bed must have an independent monitor (electrocardiograph) with an oscilloscope. This must be equipped with a pulse rate meter and a readout trigger. Each bed-monitor should be attached to a slave unit at

229

the nursing module. The slave unit should also have an oscilloscope, pulse rate meter, and readout trigger. The readout mechanism is necessary to have a recorded ECG of monitored events and is quite necessary to perform a thorough reading of the monitored ECG. The slave unit should also have an audio and visual alarm system connected to the pulse rate meter. In addition, the monitor should have at least one (and preferably two) pressure-sensitive connections for the monitoring of arterial pressure and/or wedge pressure. Pressure transducers and connector cables are also required for these systems.

The CCU should have at least two defibrillators (one for standby), an adequate supply of transvenous pacemakers, and a crash cart. The latter should contain all the drugs necessary for Emergency Cardiac Care (ECC) as well as a full supply of ventilatory adjuncts (see Chapter 11), endotracheal tubes, laryngoscopes, and cutdown sets. Bedboards should be available at every bedside. Oxygen administration and suction equipment should also be available. An IPPB machine should be handy. The CCU nurse, and her immediate aides, should receive thorough indoctrination in the use of all equipment during her initial orientation period. Continued proficiency in the use of equipment may be insured by the periodic drills mentioned in Chapter 11.

D.   STAFF

Each CCU should have a Director appointed from the medical staff. Ideally, the Director should be a cardiologist, but an interested physician with advanced training in acute cardiology is acceptable. The Director is liaison between all members of the CCU Team when problems arise. He helps decide basic CCU policies and supervises the teaching program. He decides certain treatment policies and assigns specific duties to each member of the Team. He chooses the monitoring and supportive equipment for the CCU. He may take command during emergency situations, if necessary, and serve as consultant to the attending staff.

Attending physicians who admit patients to the CCU must be proficient in basic and advanced life support and schooled in the team approach to ECC. They must be willing to sacrifice some of their therapeutic autonomy to the Team. The medical staff should have had some advanced training in treatment of the acute coronary patient. Many programs are available for such training through medical schools, hospitals, and independent organizations. The medical staff should keep themselves abreast of current techniques and approaches to the treatment of the acute coronary patient by continuing education programs. These physicians should be certified and re-certified at certain intervals for basic and advanced life support.

In teaching hospitals, which have a house staff, the intern or resident can be an important addition to the Team. However, before assuming his responsibilities on the CCU, he should have rigorous training in the policies of the CCU and be willing to work as a Team member. In many instances, the CCU nurse must be the Team leader.

The nursing staff for the CCU should be carefully selected for their training and experience in acute coronary care. They should have an orientation period and receive extensive indoctrination in acute coronary care before assuming their responsibility as CCU nurses. Emphasis should be placed on the early recognition and treatment of arrhythmias and the early recognition of other complications of acute myocardial infarction. When the CCU is combined with the ICU (as will be the case in many small hospitals), the nurse should also be knowledgeable of other life threatening complications (such as hemorrhage). She should be certified for basic and advanced life support and should receive recertification at periodic intervals.

The CCU nurse is the key to the success of this specialized unit. She will, most often, be the first member of the Team to offer basic life support, and she will be the one to start treatment of life-threatening arrhythmias. Therefore, she must have the authority to administer oxygen, start intravenous fluids, give intravenous medications, perform cardioversion in emergency situations, initiate or adjust a pacemaker, perform basic and advanced life support, and apply rotating tourniquets.

Much of this responsibility must, on occasion, be delegated to the LVN, and the latter should share training with the RN. The optimal staffing ratio is one nurse to two or three cardiac patients.

The Team will consist of other members besides those already mentioned. These may be nursing assistants, ward clerks, inhalation therapists or other paramedical personnel. Each member should be rehearsed in his duties. See Chapter 11.

E. ADMISSION & DISCHARGE POLICY

Seventy per cent of the total mortality in the CCU occurs within the first five days, and over 40% in the first 24 hours. Only 13% occurs in the third, fourth, and fifth days. The admission policy should be such that unnecessary admissions are discouraged. Because the purpose of the unit is to offer the latest treatment to the probable infarction patient, it is inevitable that a certain percentage of admissions will not prove to be infarction patients. This percentage may run as high as 60%, and this is certainly acceptable. On the other hand, the admission of a patient who by history and other findings has sustained an infarct at least 3 days prior to admission, must be questioned. The total length of stay in the CCU varies from center to center. A reasonable average stay is five days.

Admission to the CCU may come from a direct admission or from the emergency room. If the latter is the case, it is strongly recommended that certain measures be taken before the patient is taken from the ER. This would include placement of monitor electrodes and the starting of an IV. There is a high incidence of arrhythmias occurring while the patient is being transferred from the ER to the CCU.

The problem always arises, even in large CCUs, as to which patient is to be admitted when only a limited number of beds are available. There are a number of circumstances in which this situation may arise. 1) One bed is available and two patients are admitted. One patient has a chronic circulatory problem and the second is a "good risk" coronary patient. Which one is to be admitted? Several considerations come into focus with this question. Firstly, the chronic patient is not a candidate for the CCU by the very nature of his disease. In most cases, this kind of patient can be managed as well on the regular medical ward as in the CCU. Secondly, there is no such thing as a "good risk" coronary patient. Statistics have shown quite well that the clinically "good risk" coronary patient has a 9% chance of dying from his infarction. 2) The CCU is full and a patient is presented for admission. Here again, several factors must be considered. How long have the current patients been in the CCU? Have they been shown to have had infarctions? Have they stabilized, and can they be moved? Does the new patient have unequivocal evidence of infarction? In most cases, the attending staff physician will allow patients to be moved from the CCU if the situation is explained. In some cases, the CCU director must make this decision, and by written CCU policy must be given the authority to do so.

In regard to priority of admission, we should mention briefly the three classes of patients to be admitted to the CCU. Class I is the patient with unequivocal evidence of acute infarction (q waves, pain and an enzyme rise). Class II patients have pain, ST segment and T wave changes and an enzyme rise. Class III patients have pain, an abnormal ECG, and non-specific enzyme changes. The mortality rate in Classes I and II is 30%, while the mortality rate in Class III is only 3%.

F.   PROTOCOL & FORMS

A standard operating procedure is mandatory for the efficient operation of the CCU. All procedures must be clearly defined and written as such in the CCU Procedural Manual.

A Policy Manual for the CCU must define admission and discharge policy, the responsibilities of the Director, CCU nurse, admitting physician and CCU Committee. It should also indicate education and training requirements for CCU personnel. The CCU Committee should consist of the CCU Director, Nursing Director, and other department representatives having any function in the CCU.

This committee should meet at regular intervals and review the functioning of the

CCU in a retrospective and prospective manner. Policies of the CCU should be set by this committee, and full minutes should be kept of all meetings. The CCU Committee can also function as the Life Support Audit Committee (see Chapter 11).

Standard CCU Orders are an absolute necessity, and the CCU cannot function as such without them. The Orders should specify all limitations of activity, diet and fluids by mouth, vital signs, IV fluids, medications, and requested laboratory tests. They also should specify when the admitting physician is to be notified. All the above parts of the Orders can be modified by the admitting physician. The last part of the Orders should contain a section describing measures to be taken in case of emergency. Basically, this section gives the nurse legal permission to treat arrhythmias, give basic life support, and start advanced life support (see Chapter 11). This last section should be so written that it cannot be modified.

A written policy for the care and maintenance of percutaneous venous catheters should also be a part of the Procedural Manual. Nurses should be certified by the Director of the CCU in their proficiency of insertion of percutaneous venous catheters.

Nurses and physicians should be certified for their proficiency in basic and advanced life support and re-certified at appropriate intervals.

A written inspection and maintenance policy for all electrical equipment in the CCU should be a part of the Policy Manual. This should describe the responsibilities of the CCU nurse, the maintenance department, and the bio-medical engineering technician for routine maintenance and inspection of all equipment.

235

Duplicate inspection forms should be maintained on the piece of equipment and in a central file for the unit.

G.   ELECTRICAL HAZARDS

It has been estimated that between 1200 and 5000 deaths occur annually from electrocution in the CCU! Many of these deaths go unrecognized as electrical deaths. We will not go into a full discussion of the electrical principles involved, but it would be worth while to consider the meaning of macroshock and microshock. Macroshock are shocks from large amounts of electric current applied externally to the body. It takes a macroshock of 100,000 microamperes of electricity to cause ventricular fibrillation. A macroshock of 50,000 microamperes may cause much soft tissue damage and fainting, but will leave cardiac function intact. Microshock is an electric current applied directly to the myocardium. The current necessary to produce ventricular fibrillation by microshock is 20 microamperes.

The CCU patient is especially susceptible to microshock because of the instrumentation used in the CCU. The patient may have an intracardiac catheter (CVP line or PA line) or he may have a transvenous pacemaker catheter, which is even more dangerous.

Currents in the microshock range are commonly encountered in every kitchen and workshop. They are hardly felt by the victim, but the same current applied directly to the heart of the CCU patient may be fatal. The difference is due to the excellent insulating properties of the skin.

Leakage current is a minute amount of electricity that "leaks" from any electrically

236

powered piece of equipment. The presence of leakage current does not mean that the piece of equipment or the electrical connections are defective. It must be taken for granted and provisions made for its grounding. However, total elimination of leakage current is not possible, especially in more sophisticated equipment with its elaborate and complex circuitry. Current safety standards prohibit a leakage current greater than 10 microamperes (one-half the current necessary to produce ventricular fibrillation).

The danger of leakage current can be eliminated by use of proper grounding. Grounding is the key to electrical safety in the CCU. Without going into details, it should be mentioned that problems can arise if there exists a difference in the electrical potential between the separate grounds used for a single patient. For this reason, all electrical equipment used on a patient should have a common ground. Naturally, the ground should be inspected to insure its adequacy. Non-grounded plugs should never be used. This includes two-pronged plugs, cheaters, extension plugs, and defective three-pronged plugs. The latter are sometimes encased in plastic, and a defect cannot be detected except by X-ray. Certain rules of grounding can be applied to patient care:

1.   The patient should never be deliberately grounded.
2.   All appliances used on a patient should go to a common ground by a three-wire circuit.
3.   Grounding to a water pipe, neutral wire, or cable is not acceptable.
4.   Cheater plugs, extensions, or broken three-pronged plugs should never be used.
5.   Mobile equipment must be grounded before use.

6. If a patient mentions receiving a "shock" from a piece of equipment, it should not be used until it has had a thorough inspection by one knowledgeable in electric circuitry.

7. Electric beds are commonly used in modern hospitals, but their use in the CCU is to be discouraged.

Trained maintenance personnel should routinely inspect leakage currents, controls, connections, lines, plugs, fuses, and grounds of all equipment used in the CCU. An inspection schedule should be established for all equipment. Recommendations for such a schedule are described in Circulation, 44: A-237, 1971.

(SAMPLE)

CORONARY CARE ORDERS

ACTIVITY

1. Bed rest. Head of bed to be elevated to position of comfort.
2. Bed bath. Complete care by nurse. May shave male patient PRN.
3. Bedside commode if free of shock. Assist to avoid lifting of trunk, walking, or any but minimal effort.
4. Elastic thigh-length stockings to legs. Remove for 30 minutes every 4 hours during day.
5. Passive exercises of legs when stockings are changed every 4 hours during day.
6. No smoking.
7. Use of TV and radio regulated by nurse.
8. Visiting to be regulated by nurse. Immediate family only, limited to a small number of visitors at any time and for short intervals.
9. Weigh daily before breakfast. May stand if free of pain or shock.
10. _____

DIET & FLUIDS

1. Clear liquids for first 24 hours, progressing to controlled fat diet plan as tolerated. 1200 calories, 1 gm sodium. No iced liquids.
2. Record intake and output.
3. Encourage oral fluids.
4. _____

VITAL SIGNS (BP, P, R, T, CVP, Urine output)

1. Vital signs every ½ hour until stable, then every hour times six, then every 2 hours. Omit BP when patient is sleeping if pulse is strong, rate normal & stable.

2. Oral temperature QID. Rectal temperature if condition prevents accurate oral temp.
3. Rhythm strips every 2-4 hours as indicated, with regular rhythm. More frequently with arrhythmia.
4. Monitor patient with oscilloscope. Heart rate meter set at 60 and 110.
5. Foley catheter to volumetric device. Measure urine volume every hour during first 24 hours.
6. _____

IV FLUIDS

1. 1000cc 5% D/W with Heparin 1000 units IV. Give at rate of 15 micro-drops/min.
2. Nurse may start IV.
3. If plastic catheter is used, prepare with surgical skin preparation and daily dressing as per policy regarding care of percutaneous venous catheters.
4. _____

MEDICATIONS

1. Oxygen at 5-6 L/min by nasal cannula, or 8 L/min with plastic mask or rebreathing mask. Use humidifier bottle. Use for cardiac pain, dyspnea, cyanosis or shock.
2. Surfak 240 mg BID, or_____
3. Meprobamate 200 mg QID, or_____
4. Chloral Hydrate 1 gm hs PRN sleep, rep 500 mg PRN, or_____
5. Morphine sulfate 3 mg every 5 to 30 minutes IV for cardiac pain, or Demerol 50 mg IV every 4 hours for cardiac pain, or_____
6. Atropine 0.5 mg IV for abrupt onset of bradycardia (50/min) when physician is not immediately available. Rate to be determined by sinus or nodal rhythm only (when possible).
7. NO INTRAMUSCULAR MEDICATIONS.
8. _____

LABORATORY

.1. First Day
   CBC, urinalysis, VDRL, cholesterol, fasting blood sugar, triglycerides (with fractions), BUN, uric acid, serum Na, K, HCO_3, Cl, Ca, PO_4, creatinine, bilirubin, CPK, LDH, SGOT.
2. Second Day
   CPK, LDH, SGOT, pro-time.
3. Third Day
   Creatinine, CPK, CBC.
4. Fourth Day
   LDH, SGOT.
5. 12-lead electrocardiogram on admission, 2nd day and 4th day.
6. Portable chest X-ray 1st or 2nd day.
7. _____

CALL ADMITTING PHYSICIAN IF

1. Systolic BP is below 90 or above 180 mmHg.
2. Heart rate below 60 or above 110.
3. Urine output below 25 cc/hour.
4. Central venous pressure below 5 or above 15 cm water.
5. Wedge pressure above 14 mmHg.
6. Any unusual arrhythmia. Take rhythm strip.
7. Patient complains of persistent chest pain, unusual anxiety, dyspnea, or other problems.
8. _____

CARDIAC EMERGENCY

Arrhythmias which are life-threatening include:

1. Premature Ventricular Contractions (PVCs) when:
   a. Any occur during the first 4 hours following an infarction.
   b. They occur at a rate of 5 per minute or more.
   c. They are multifocal.
   d. They occur in pairs or runs.
   e. They occur on the T wave.

241

(SAMPLE)

Treatment of PVCs
1. Lidocaine 50 mg bolus IV stat, may repeat in one minute if necessary.
2. Follow with 500 cc 5% D/W containing 2 gms Lidocaine and run at rate of 1 mg/min (15 micro-drops/min.) May increase to maximum of 4 mg/min (60 micro-drops/min) if necessary to keep PVCs less than 5 per minute.
3. Notify physician to obtain additional Lidocaine orders.
4. Do not give Lidocaine with complete Heart Block.

Note: Ventricular ectopic beats which are associated with a bradycardia or appear to be escape beats are best treated with Atropine 0.5 to 1 mg IV or other methods to increase the heart beat.

2. Ventricular Tachycardia
Treatment of VT
1. If the patient is alert and has a palpable pulse give Lidocaine as detailed above. Alert physician.
2. If the patient is unconscious or has no palpable carotid pulse administer immediately DC countershock at 400 Watt seconds. Summon physician.

PROCEDURE FOLLOWING CARDIAC ARREST

1. Ventricular Fibrillation
1. Heart rate alarm sounds. Nurse to bedside. Check monitor for false alarm, ventricular fibrillation or cardiac standstill (asystole).
2. Check patient: appearance, airway, carotid pulse, pupils to confirm arrest.
3. Deliver precordial thump. Sound alarm.
4. Place bed in flat position, remove pillow, open airway.
5. Defibrillate at 400 Watt seconds, if no physician present. Rep X 1 PRN.

(SAMPLE)

6. Place board under patient and start CPR.
   A. Open airway.
   B. Breathe for patient.
   C. Circulate for patient with closed-chest cardiac compression.
7. Repeat defibrillation at 400 Watt seconds if fibrillation persists.
8. Continue to ventilate lungs and compress chest without interruption until physician and rest of team arrives.
9. Sodium bicarbonate 44 mEq IV for every 10 minutes of arrest for two doses. Record exact time given.
10. Lidocaine (by the method above) to suppress ventricular irritability.
11. Epinephrine 1 mg (1 cc of 1:1000) IV; dilute to 10 cc in water or saline and give every five minutes of arrest.

2. Ventricular Standstill (Asystole)

1. Heart rate alarm sounds. Nurse to bedside. Check monitor for false alarm, ventricular fibrillation of cardiac standstill (asystole).
2. Check patient: appearance, airway, carotid pulse, pupils to confirm arrest.
3. Deliver precordial thump. Sound alarm.
4. Place bed in flat position, remove pillow, open airway.
5. Turn on pacemaker, if one in place.
6. Place board under patient and start CPR.
   A. Open airway.
   B. Breathe for patient.
   C. Circulate for patient with closed-chest cardiac compression.
7. Continue to ventilate lungs and compress chest without interruption until physician and rest of team arrives.
8. Epinephrine STAT in dose noted above.
9. Sodium bicarbonate as described above.

THESE ORDERS ARE IN EFFECT UNLESS OTHER ORDERS ARE WRITTEN BY THE ATTENDING PHYSICIAN. CARDIAC EMERGENCY ORDERS CANNOT BE MODIFIED.

Date _____   _____
                              Physician's Signature

The following are orders which can be
used for patients who are being transferred
out of the CCU.

(SAMPLE)

CCU INTERMEDIARY ORDERS

1. BRP, bedbath.
2. Weigh daily.
3. Regular low salt diet, low cholesterol diet, lipoprotein diet. (Indicate
   which desired.)
4. BP, P, R, T QID.
5. Rhythm strip daily.
6. Surfak 240 mg daily.
7. Analgesic_____
8. Hypnotic_____
9. Continue routine CCU lab until
   finished.
10. Continue antiembolic hose. Instruct
    patient in removing every 4 hours.
11. DC I & O
12. DC Foley catheter
13. DC IV
14. _____
15. _____

CHAPTER 13

PREVENTIONS AND THE FUTURE

When we talk about preventing heart
attacks, we are talking about the prevention
of two separate and sometimes distinct syndromes — arteriosclerotic heart disease and
myocardial infarction. The first problem
that must be solved, if we are to prevent
these two syndromes, is to identify those
individuals to which they might occur.

A great many studies have been done
in an attempt to identify the factors which
lead to coronary artery disease. The most
famous of these was the Framingham Study,
in which an entire town was studied for many
years. From this study, and others, research-
ers have derived a list of risk factors. The
presence of a risk factor is supposed to enhance the possibility of an individual developing arteriosclerotic heart disease.

A.   RISK FACTORS

The first two risk factors are those
over which we have no control — age and
sex. In any age group, the incidence of ASHD
is higher in males than in females. Before the
menopause, the difference is sizable. After
the menopause, females tend to become more
susceptible to ASHD but still lag far behind
males. Age is a rather obvious factor — the
older one becomes, the more likely they are
to suffer from ASHD.

Diet. It has been shown by numerous
studies that patients with hypercholesterol-
emia and/or hyperlipoproteinemia (as measured by serum triglyceride level) have a
higher incidence of ASHD. It is still unclear
whether these elevated levels of fats represent

245

dietary patterns or metabolic abnormalities. However, when such an elevation is discovered, it is common practice to counsel the patient on dietary corrective measures, in hope of bringing the level back to normal. Cholesterol control diets and diets to control one or more of the five lipoprotein fractions are commonly used in clinical practice. These diets are often combined with clofibrate (Atromid-S), a drug used to lower certain blood lipids.

Hypernutrition, obesity, is a risk factor by itself, and is an additive cause of hypertension and diabetes mellitus.

Hypertension, which goes uncontrolled, is a definite risk factor, and the degree of risk increases in proportion to the amount of hypertension.

Cigarette smoking is a risk factor that has received a great deal of publicity. It seems that the moderate or heavy smoker has a much higher risk of ASHD than the non-smoker or light smoker. It has also been shown, that if a smoker gives up the habit, his risk returns toward normal (but not to normal).

The above risk factors are additive in their combined effects.

Diabetes mellitus and asymptomatic hyperglycemia are other risk factors and seem to be independent from the above factors.

Exercise habits also seem to be independent of the above factors. Light to moderate exercise of the type that enhances cardiopulmonary fitness seems to offer some protection from ASHD. A sedentary life style is a risk factor.

A resting tachycardia and a family history of coronary artery disease are risk factors over which we have no control. Of course, a past personal history of abnormal electrocardiograms is an obvious risk factor.

The American Heart Association has prepared a booklet, "Coronary Risk Handbook", which details, in table form, the impact of each risk factor on an individual's chance of developing coronary artery disease. The major variables in this booklet are the risk factors over which the individual has some control: smoking, diet (cholesterol), blood pressure, and abnormal glucose tolerance.

The risk factor concept in explaining coronary artery disease is not without controversy. The major point of dissension is the fact that for every study showing that the presence of any one of the risk factors leads to a higher incidence of ASHD, there is another study to show that this is not the case. For instance, it has been shown that in a group of people with a very high cholesterol diet, there is an increased rate of coronary artery disease. In another group of people, with an equally high cholesterol diet, there is a low rate of ASHD. The same is true of nearly all the risk factors. By using risk factor prediction, we can account for only about 50% of the cases of ASHD.

B.   THE TYPE A PERSONALITY

Two San Francisco cardiologists, Meyer Friedman and Ray Rosenman have come up with another theory for the etiology of ASHD. They feel that nearly all patients suffering an acute myocardial infarction belong to what they define as the Type A personality. A Type A personality is an individual with a "hurry-up sickness". These people have a malignant compulsion to strive and to achieve as much as possible in as little time as possible. They are impatient, usually hostile, and will not be "out-done". These people are not neurotics, nor do they appear to be sick. They may be executives, but may also be mechanics or street-sweepers. They don't know how to relax and enjoy life, but they don't complain of being sick.

These people are seldom seen by a psychiatrist, but may be seen by an internist or general practitioner. It is up to this physician to identify the Type A and attempt to modify his behavior. Doctors Friedman and Rosenman feel that this can be done and without the necessity of lengthy psychoanalysis. They describe this process in their book, Type A Behavior and Your Heart.

These doctors present impressive statistical data to back up their theory. They have also found that the Type A man has an increased secretion of catecholamines (norepinephrine and VMA), high fasting levels of triglycerides, betalipoproteins, and cholesterol, and marked slowing of fat clearing from the blood. Their blood also clots faster. All of these findings are reversed when the Type A man modifies his behavior toward normal.

The following signs are used to identify the Type A personality: 1) chronic sense of time urgency, 2) free-floating hostility (must win at any game; must win any argument), 3) must do things faster, 4) explosive speech pattern, walks rapidly, eats rapidly, nervous habits, 5) chronically impatient, 6) mind always busy, 7) can converse only on topics that interest him, 8) feels guilty when relaxing, 9) no time for doing things because time is spent in acquiring things.

The Type B man is never impatient, hostile, and never suffers from a sense of time urgency. He also has a normal cholesterol.

248

Friedman and Rosenman have devised a "Mini-manual" for self-improvement of the Type A personality. It consists firstly of self-appraisal. Secondly, there are recommendations for establishing a new life style, and finally, they describe measures to combat the "hurry-up sickness". The reader is referred to their book for a complete discussion of these.

It may be many years before we are able to say with absolute assurance that Factor X or Factor Y causes ASHD. Meanwhile, we must muddle along with what knowledge we do have. In clinical practice, even though the question of risk factors is entirely unsettled, we still try to limit them as much as possible. An obese patient is encouraged to reduce. A smoker is advised to stop. Hypertension and diabetes are controlled. A diet of unsaturated fats is recommended, as is a moderate exercise program. In addition, the Type A personality is identified and counseled to change his ways. Whether we are really minimizing the risks of ASHD by this approach, only time will tell. At any rate, it seems certain that we can do no harm to the patient by this type of counseling.

C.   PREVENTION OF ACUTE INFARCTIONS

The approach to the prevention of acute myocardial infarction is somewhat different. This group is presumably made up of those with ASHD and those with no demonstrable ASHD. The latter are those who meet sudden death from spasm-induced ventricular fibrillation. A few patients in this group will have been diagnosed by arteriography and placed on antispasmodics. There seems little that can be done at the present time for the remainder. In the group of patients with ASHD there is much that can be done.

249

If the patient with suspicious chest pain has a normal resting electrocardiogram, a stress electrocardiogram should be done. If this is abnormal, coronary arteriograms can be performed. If major vessel disease is detected, a saphenous vein by-pass procedure can be performed with little operative mortality in experienced hands.

The stress or exercise ECG is recommended as routine follow-up at 3, 6, and 12 months following an infarct to access the activity allowable for the patient. It is also indicated for patients with anginal-type chest pain, but with a normal resting ECG. It is also used for routine cardiac evaluation for selected patients.

During the exercise ECG, the patients are put on a treadmill and their ECG monitored, while their heart rate is brought up to a predicted value (according to age and sex). The test is terminated when 1) they reach the predicted heart rate with no significant ECG changes or 2) there is a 1 mm or more elevation or depression of the ST segment. Other ECG changes (such as PVCs) do not necessarily mean ischemia. (A change in the ST segment of 3 to 4 mm usually means proximal disease of the left coronary artery or its two major branches.)

The exercise ECG is contraindicated in patients with crescendo angina (pre-infarction angina) or in patients with ECG evidence of ischemic heart disease, or in patients with congestive heart failure. It should never be done on an unstable patient. It must be done with great care by one experienced in its use. Treatment for sinus bradycardia and ventricular ectopy should be immediately available.

The patient with positive findings on the exercise ECG should be referred for cor-

250

onary arteriography. This procedure should also be done on those patients who have survived an infarction.

In coronary arteriography, a catheter is fed into a peripheral artery (usually the femoral or brachial) up to the coronary ostia. The catheter is then advanced into each of the two major vessels and radiopaque dye injected. X-ray movies are then taken as the dye perfuses the coronary circulation. Obstructive lesions are precisely identified and located by this procedure. During the same procedure, a catheter is advanced into the left ventricle and then the left atrium, and dye injected. This shows the competency of the aortic and mitral valves and the contractile efficiency of the chambers. Septal defects can also be detected. Oxygen saturation and pressures in each chamber can be measured, and the cardiac output can be directly measured by the dye dilution technique.

The one-year mortality for various kinds of vessel disease due to acute myocardial infarction was discussed in Chapter 5. The operative mortality for saphenous vein by-pass is less than 4% in most centers. Candidates for this procedure are those with demonstrated proximal vessel disease, especially left-sided disease. The one-year mortality rate for main left coronary artery disease is 10-15%. A lesion of the anterior descending branch of the left coronary artery is so ominous it is called the "widowmaker" lesion.

In one group of patients, the saphenous vein by-pass is sometimes done on an emergency basis. This is the group with so-called pre-infarction angina (crescendo angina, unstable angina). These are usually people with a long history of stable angina who have noticed a sudden increase in the chest pain which is not controlled by the usual means. In addition, there are ECG changes during the spells of chest pain, but no enzyme changes. These spells of chest pain may be controlled with conservative management, but the 18-month mortality in the group is 20%.

As was mentioned in an earlier Chapter, surgery offers definitive treatment for acute mitral insufficiency and acute septal perforation following an infarct. The balloon pump is used until the patient is ready for surgery (ideally, six weeks, if the patient can be stabilized). The balloon pump also offers assistance to the patient in cardiogenic shock and the patient with an extending infarct. It improves coronary perfusion and decreases the after-load on the heart.

D.   THE FUTURE

In the future, we may look forward to many new mechanical assists to cardiac function. Research is now being done on several types of mechanical hearts, and perhaps the day will come when a small atomic-powered pump will replace the heart in failure or shock. Heart transplantation has been a moderate success. Further research is currently being done on this procedure, and in a few years, this might prove to be very fruitful.

We might look forward to drugs which will prevent arteriosclerosis and to other drugs which will reverse the processes of arteriosclerosis. We may also look forward to drugs which will be more useful and less dangerous for the treatment of the medical complications of acute infarction. A recent recommendation by one cardiologist is that ASHD patients with a known propensity to PVCs carry with them at all times, a self-injectable ampoule of Lidocaine.

As surgical techniques are advanced and perfected, we will also see a lower mortality in surgical complications. Along with this, must go better methods of diagnosing occult or early complications. Computer analysis offers one possible adjunct to this approach.

In the future, when the recommendations of the National Conference on Standards for CPR and ECG become a fact, mobile life support units will be readily available in every community and at every large public gathering. Perhaps by that time, many lay people will be trained in basic life support. With prompt basic life support, many thousands of people could be saved each year. With the use of basic in-ambulance telemetry, life threatening arrhythmias could be diagnosed, treated, and reversed. Advanced life support will be practiced by the mobile life support units. All of this will take time.

INDEX

A

Acetazolamide   135
Acid-Base Balance   122, 128, 146
Acidity, blood   122
  measurement of   123
Acidosis 74, 122, 124, 128
  compensated   127
  lactic   122, 143
  metabolic   126, 135
  mixed   127
  respiratory 37, 126, 134
  transmembrane potential
  effect on   37
Action potential 35, 36
Adrenergic blocking
  agents   178
ADH   136
Airway   191, 195, 199
  Adjuncts   199, 214
  Esophageal obturator   214
  Head-tilt method   191, 197
  Jaw-thrust method   191
Akinesis, ventricular   118
Aldosterone   136, 137
Alkalosis   124, 128
  Metabolic   126, 135, 154
  Respiratory   126, 134
Alpha Adrenergic Stimu-
  lation   174, 175
Antiarrhythmia drugs   161,
  163, 171-172, 179-182
  Type I   161, 162, 171
  Type II   165, 166, 172
Ammonium ion   134
Aneurysm, ventricular   119
Angiotensin   137, 182
Anticoagulants   148, 149
  in pulmonary embolism   120

A (cont'd)

Antidiuretic hormone   136
Arrest – see Cardiac
Arrhythmias   84
  Bradyarrhythmias   91
  Electrical failure   101
  Electrical instability   85
  Pump failure   104
Arteriography, coronary   251
Arterioles, precapillary   30
Arteriosclerosis   70, 71, 72
Arteriosclerotic heart
  disease   69
  mortality   69
Artery, carotid   27
  coronary
    blood flow 11
    left   8, 10, 11, 42
      anterior descending
      branch   8, 10
      circumflex branch
        8, 10, 11, 41
    right   8, 10, 11, 42
      posterior descending
      branch 8, 10, 41
    spasm of   73
  pulmonary   2, 3, 6
Artificial circulation   190
Artificial ventilation   190
Atherosclerosis   71, 72
Atrial fibrillation   98, 100
Atrial flutter   56, 97, 100
Atrioventricular node – see
  AV node
Atrium, left   1, 3, 6, 14, 16, 17
Atrium, right   1, 2, 6, 14, 16
Atrium, hypertrophy   54
Atropine   37, 93, 167, 182, 214

260